Praise for
Your Health is in Your Hands

"Jim Jordan presents a clear, concise scientific and holistic approach to health. His experience speaks for itself and the facts are documented, easy to understand and to the point. His message delivers the goods without all the fluff."

-Dr. Timothy March, DC

"Jim Jordan's approach to health and healing is unique from other practitioners in the field of Health and Wellness. He has been down the very long path of severe chronic illness and found his way to a high level of wellness through trial and error, and applied intelligence. Jim applies this accumulated wisdom and understanding of the body, mind and spirit in his practice and offers a practical and efficient way to expedite the self healing process for his clients. Jim's track record speaks for itself in his success…"

-Lee Patrick Hanks, Health Consultant

Jim Jordan has written an exceptional book on the primary, underlying factors that prevent people from achieving ideal health. This is a wake-up call for anyone serious about reclaiming their health through the use of diet, nutrition, detoxification, right attitude and healthy lifestyle. He writes from not only his clinical experience, but also from his personal health journey. This is a very eye-opening book.

-Michael McEvoy, FDN, CNC, CMTA

"Herein lie the keys to vibrant health! Jim Jordan lays out the fundamentals to optimal health. He dispels myths and tells the truth that he has proved through the healing of his own chronic fatigue and in his work with countless health seekers over the past 25 years. Read it, then follow it to reclaim and enhance your own health."

-Michael Mendribil, ND

Your Health is in Your Hands

The Three Reasons You're Not Well and What to do About It

By James D. Jordan, CNC, JD

©2014 Create Vibrant Health All rights reserved. Printed in USA. The content of this book is protected by copyright. Reproduction of the content, whether in whole or part, is prohibited without the prior written consent of Create Vibrant Health.

Cover designed by Caitlin Mezger-Sieg and Jacquelene Ambrose

This book is designed to assist you in finding greater health and quality of life. It is not meant to diagnose, treat or replace any necessary medical care. Each person and situation is unique. If you are under the care of a health professional, then check with them before starting any activity mentioned in this book that could impact your condition.

All names of clients used in this book are fictitious but the stories are true.

Dedication

I have two primary teachers to thank for the information I will share with you in this book, Jim Lane and Michael Coyle. These remarkable men taught me that health is a result of multiple factors. They taught me that each person must learn about the underlying causes of their health issues and address the areas which have the biggest impact on bringing about a transformation in one's health.

Jim trained me in live blood cell analysis and how to use this technology as a teaching tool to educate and motivate people to take responsibility for their own health. He is a man of enormous patience, intelligence and heart. Michael gave me the vision of teaching the underlying causation paradigm on a broader scale by training groups of healthcare practitioners in live blood cell analysis. Both men's faith and confidence in me have given me the strength and encouragement to continue teaching people to look to the underlying causes of health problems as opposed to treating symptoms.

I've been very fortunate to find leading edge teachers, new modalities and healthcare products that continue to advance my knowledge and understanding of health and how we can increase our vitality at any age. I decided to write and publish this book to reach more people with the often overlooked underlying causes of chronic health problems and the most practical solutions to address these causes. Consider this knowledge to be the foundation upon which to build your house of health.

April, 2014
Ashland, Oregon

Table of Contents

Introduction 1
Chapter 1: My Personal Health Journey 5
Chapter 2: Introduction to the Underlying
            Causation Paradigm 11
Chapter 3: Nutrient Deficiencies 13
       A.   Fundamental Principles of Diet
           and Nutrition 18
       B.   Common Nutrient Deficiencies 27
Chapter 4: Toxicity 38
       A.   Chemicals 42
       B.   Heavy Metals 51
       C.   Radiation 61
Chapter 5: Stress 66
       A.   The Impact of Stress 67
       B.   Adopting a Wellness Mindset 70
       C.   Letting Go of the Past 74
Chapter 6: Common Mistakes 78
Chapter 7: Frequently Asked Questions 82
Conclusion 88
Addendum A: Resource Guide 91
Addendum B: Vitamins 97
Addendum C: Minerals 101
Addendum D: Detoxification Program 104
Forms and Surveys: Daily Diet Diary 108
Toxicity Survey 109
Stress Survey 113

Acknowledgments

I want to acknowledge my mother, Claudine Jordan, and my father, Luis Jordan, for their support over the years in helping me recover my health and launch my career in natural healing. I want to acknowledge my partner, Jewel Baldwin, for her belief in me and for her assistance in editing the book. I also wish to thank Kristina Royce for her editorial assistance.

Introduction

> *"The first step in natural healing is responsibility. Natural healing is about taking control of your life and being responsible for everything that goes in and out of your body, mind and spirit."*
>
> *- Richard Schulze, Master Herbalist*

Why is it that so many people are suffering from chronic health problems? Each of us knows people of all ages with chronic health problems, some with multiple conditions. Most of these health issues were rare occurrences two or more decades ago. Today, the following chronic health conditions are on the rise: diabetes, obesity, chronic fatigue syndrome, attention deficit disorder, attention deficit hyperactivity disorder, autism, auto-immune conditions, depression, insomnia, heart disease, asthma and other chronic respiratory conditions, irritable bowel syndrome, hypothyroidism, hormone imbalances and infertility.

According to a July 2009 report published in *Clinical Laboratory News,* chronic illness is on the rise in virtually every category. Currently, more than 133 million Americans (45% of the population) have at least one chronic condition and 26% have multiple chronic conditions. Chronic disease is currently the leading cause of all death and disability in the United States, responsible for 70% of all deaths.

If this trend continues, by 2023, the picture worsens considerably with a more than 50% increase projected in cases of cancer, mental disorders and diabetes and more than 40% increase in heart disease. Hypertension and pulmonary conditions are expected to rise by more than 30% and incidences of stroke by more than 25%.

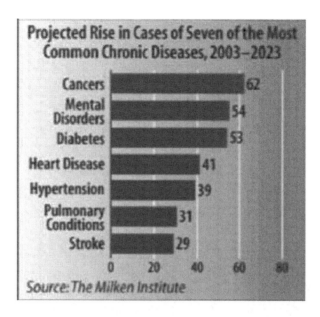

Health Decline in Children

The health of our children is an excellent barometer of the overall decline in the quality of health in the United States. Attention Deficit Hyperactivity Disorder (ADHD) is reaching epidemic levels according to a study from the Center for Disease Control. The study showed 20% of American boys age 11 had been diagnosed with ADHD at some point in their lives and 13.3% of those boys are being medicated for ADHD. But it gets worse. According to the CDC's study, the percentage of U.S. children between the ages of 4 and 17 years who have been labeled with the diagnosis, rose to a mind-boggling 42% between 2003 and 2011.

One of the most worrisome trends is the increase in childhood obesity, which has tripled in the U.S. over the past two decades resulting in the quadrupling of childhood chronic diseases in the past four decades. Due to this increase in childhood obesity, the next generation of Americans is at a greater risk for developing chronic diseases of all kinds.

Introduction

A special themed issue of The Journal of the American Medical Association (JAMA), published in June of 2007, was devoted to chronic childhood illness. The Journal defined chronic illness as any debilitating illness that lasts a year or more past diagnosis. In fact, a number of new studies suggest that the health of America's children is getting worse, not better.

Some of the findings:

- According to the analysis by James Perrin, M.D., Director of the Center for Child and Adolescent Health Policy, more than 7% of U.S. children and youth were hampered in their daily activities by an illness that lasted three months or longer in 2004, compared to just 1.8% of children in 1960.
- Chronic conditions now affect 15% to 18% of children and teens, and even those estimates may not fully account for obesity and mental health problems.
- The "big three" chronic health conditions for kids are: obesity, which affected 5% of American children in the early 1970's, and 18% of children today; asthma, 9% prevalence, nearly doubled from the 1980's; as well as attention deficit hyperactivity disorder.

This persistent decline in the health of our children is leading us to an evermore unhealthy adult population. One of the reasons for this overall decline in health is that the primary solution provided by conventional medicine is to treat symptoms with medications, and to treat the side effects of those medications with more medications. There is virtually no discussion of the underlying causes of this explosion of chronic health problems. To make matters worse, there is little or no consideration to the compounding negative effect of multiple underlying causes.

We have been socially conditioned to believe that our genetics, the natural aging process and the random exposure to pathogens are the primary factors affecting our health. We are told to take statin drugs to prevent heart disease, and flu vaccines to keep us healthy in the winter. We are also told that children and adults should take medications such as Ritalin and Prozac to treat health issues such as ADD, ADHD and depression. Is this the best conventional medicine can offer us?

This health crisis is not just about people with medically recognized diseases. Over time, we have been slowly but surely lowering our standards for what it means to be healthy. By conventional medical standards, you are considered healthy as long as you are not diagnosed with a disease. A more accurate definition of good health would include a strong immune system, the ability to adapt during stressful periods, as well as a consistent experience of vitality and mental clarity.

Since 1997, I have seen literally thousands of blood chemistries and other lab tests for patients who had "normal" numbers by conventional standards, yet many of these patients were very unhealthy. There is a vast difference between the pathological interpretation of lab tests and an optimal function interpretation of the exact same lab tests. To be in the "normal range" does not mean you are experiencing vibrant health.

Health is not just the absence of "disease" or the lack of major aggravating symptoms. Being healthy includes having vitality, a strong body and sharp mind; optimal organ function and hormone levels; and a strong digestive system. True health also includes the ability to rest and to recover quickly from stressful periods in life, and to bounce back from injuries and other health setbacks.

Chapter 1

My Personal Health Journey

I suffered from serious health challenges at two different times in my life. When I was two years old, I had severe colitis and chronic digestive disorders. My mother sought answers from the conventional medical doctors, but to no avail. After several years of searching for a solution, she finally came across a doctor who told her that I was allergic to milk and wheat. When those foods were eliminated from my diet, my health recovered. For the remainder of my childhood and teenage years, I was healthy, athletic and productive.

However, by my third year of college, I began to develop chronic headaches and indigestion. I drank a lot of beer and ate poorly during the first two years of college. I suffered from chronic insomnia and depression, even though I still was able to function relatively well. It was in the summer of 1984, between my second and third years of law school, that my health started to deteriorate rapidly. This decline in health began with a series of urinary tract infections and was followed by chronic headaches, fatigue and depression all of which plagued me the entire summer.

Over the next few years my diagnosis included:

- chronic fatigue syndrome
- heavy metal poisoning, including mercury and nickel toxicity
- systemic candida infection
- Epstein-Barr virus
- Cytomegalovirus

- chronic constipation (to the point where I needed to have a colonic in order to eliminate)
- multiple chemical sensitivities and dozens of food and inhalant allergies
- depression

Basically, I felt like I had the flu all the time. At a time when my friends were starting careers, getting married and starting families, I spent most of my twenties going to endless doctors' offices trying to understand why I felt so lousy.

All my conventional lab tests were in the "normal" range. Meanwhile, I felt horrible. I suffered from exhaustion, chronic infections, chronic headaches and insomnia. Doctors told me I should see a psychiatrist because they believed that with "normal" test results, all my problems must be in my head. After seeing a psychiatrist for several weeks, I quickly realized that this would not solve my health problems.

By the early fall of 1984, I not only lost my job as a law clerk, but I had to withdraw from law school at the beginning of my third year. During that year, I began a journey that would take me six years before my health was fully restored. Despite returning to complete law school, passing the Illinois bar exam and practicing law off and on for several years, my health issues continued to plague me throughout my 20s. Numerous times my health crashed and I had to take extended leaves of absence, even from my part-time jobs.

Fortunately, I had tremendous support from my family. I was able to keep my mind open to investigating healing modalities which, early in my illness, I would have never considered valid. During the years of my health struggles, while I followed leads and possibilities, I never had a deep understanding of the cumulative effect of multiple underlying causes of illness and how these factors impacted my health. I often felt like I was flying blind. It was only in hindsight that I understood that my recovery was a result of a combination of many factors.

In the depth of my six-year illness, I went to see a Chinese doctor in Chinatown on the near south side of Chicago. Dr. Gua didn't speak a word of English and had his granddaughter translate for me. He asked me what was wrong with me. I proceeded to repeat the long diagnosis I had developed over the past few years, which included: candida, heavy metal toxicity, viruses, chronic fatigue syndrome, etc. He listened to me and shook his head. "No, no," he said, "these are not your problems. You are just **not** healthy. When you are healthy you cannot be sick."

I paused and let his words sink in. Like a lightning bolt, it hit me that my focus had been on my problems the whole time. This understanding was a turning point for me. Over the next year my approach to healing radically shifted. I gave up all labels to my health condition and put my attention 100% on nourishing and strengthening my body, mind and spirit.

By age 28, I started an ascent from the deepest suffering I had ever experienced in my life to levels of well being I could not have previously imagined. My moods and energy dramatically improved; my ability to digest and assimilate nutrition improved, and my overall vitality was restored. Most importantly, I had faith again in life and in myself.

At various times during the years to come I had minor setbacks, but each time, when I applied a more holistic understanding of health, I was able to restore my health and vitality. I learned that whenever I felt less than optimal, I should always look to the underlying causes of why I did not feel well.

My return to health had three stages. First, I rejected things that were obviously not working for me. Second, I opened my mind to all reasonable therapies, diets and healing modalities, which could increase my vitality and strength and at the same time had no toxic side effects. Finally, I found meaning to my life, which was to get well and help others get well.

From Lawyer to Nutritional Consultant and Health Educator

In 1989, with vastly improved health, I was able to return full-time to work as a lawyer, but I was already thinking of a new career. I found myself giving nutrition and health advice to my law partner, family, friends and some of my legal clients. I also started a sideline business selling food-based Chinese herbs, which had played a significant role in my healing. I found myself giving talks at various venues in the Chicago area and eventually started a small sideline nutrition coaching practice.

One of my first nutrition clients was a personal injury client who had gained an enormous amount of weight since her automobile accident. She said she had gained this weight despite doing everything possible to lose weight. She had cut back on her calories and was eating only one or two meals a day. Her diet consisted of macaroni and cheese and an occasional salad.

I designed a healthy diet plan for her which included: three healthy meals a day, vegetables with each meal, healthy choices for protein, like salmon and naturally raised chicken, some fruit and healthy fatty foods like avocados and olive oil. After a couple of months on this program my client lost over 20 pounds of unhealthy fat even though she had substantially increased her caloric intake. Gaining unhealthy weight is often a result of a metabolic imbalance that can only be corrected with good nutrition not through calorie restriction.

For the first time as an adult I had a vision of a career that I would enjoy and I knew would make a difference for people. However, it took another six years before I had sufficient training and confidence to make a successful transition from law to natural healing.

By 1993, I had left my law practice and moved away from Chicago to start a four-year journey and seek a new life. In the back of mind during this four-year journey was the sense that someday I would enter the field of natural healing. My opportunity came after moving to Boulder, Colorado in 1994. I started working in the field of nutritional supplement sales for several different companies and giving talks to small groups of people.

In the summer of 1996, in Boulder, Colorado, I met Jim Lane, a man who would change my life forever. Within six months, I had moved back to Chicago to begin an intensive study of live blood cell analysis (LBCA) with Jim Lane as my mentor. Live Blood Cell analysis is a system designed to study blood using a microscope with a video camera hooked up to a viewing monitor. What excited me about LBCA was that it allowed the client to view their blood in real time and to see how toxins and nutrient deficiencies impact their health.

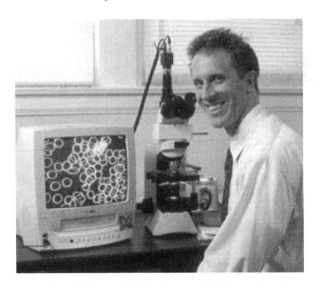

My early days with the microscope in the year 2000

Jim Lane and my other Live Blood Cell Analysis mentor, Michael Coyle, both taught me that health problems are the result of multiple dietary, environmental and psycho-emotional factors. It is the synergy and accumulation of these factors over time, which ultimately manifest in a unique way depending upon one's weaknesses and vulnerabilities.

Since 1996, I studied many modalities of natural healing and assessment tools including: Reiki energy healing, live and dry blood cell analysis, hair tissue mineral analysis, quantum reflex analysis, metabolic typing and more. In 1998, I received my national certification as a Certified Nutritional Consultant from the American Association of Nutritional Consultants. I worked as a nutritional consultant and live blood cell microscope technician at Dr. Joseph Mercola's Optimal Wellness Center from 2000 to 2004. I've had my own nutrition and wellness practice since 1997, and I have trained dozens of health care professionals in live blood cell microscopy. Over the past 17 years, I've trained both health care practitioners and natural health enthusiasts to work as nutrition and wellness coaches.

What I have discovered over the years is that the basic underlying causes of chronic health problems have not changed since my health collapsed in 1984. In each private session with a client and in my training seminars, I review these same causes over and over again. There are variations in approaches to address these underlying causes, but the causes remain the same. The knowledge of the underlying causation paradigm is the first step in helping you and your loved ones recover from any chronic illness and maintain higher levels of health and vitality for the rest of your life.

Chapter 2

The Underlying Causation of Illness Paradigm

Your health issues, the process of aging, and most of your physical and emotional suffering are caused primarily by these three factors:

- Nutrient Deficiencies
- Toxicity
- Stress

In order to maximize your chance of living a vibrant and healthy life, you must understand how these causes operate, and you must also understand how to incorporate practical tools and strategies to address these causes.

Whether your issue is chronic fatigue, high blood pressure, obesity, memory loss, depression, hypothyroidism, chronic pain, Irritable Bowel Syndrome, asthma, debilitating allergies, ADD/ADHD or just aging faster than you'd like, understanding the **Underlying Causation Paradigm** (UCP) is the starting point for you to improve your health. If you are a parent and you want to help your children have the healthiest lives they can, this information is the foundation of a knowledge base that you can build on for years to come.

For every individual, the combination of nutrient deficiencies, toxins and stresses will be unique and each person will have a unique way to resolve these issues. For example, if you're struggling with depression and fatigue, you may need to identify the primary toxicities you have been exposed to and understand which nutrients you may need to increase.

For another individual, also suffering from depression and fatigue, the solution may be entirely different. This person may need to reduce exposure to electro-magnetic radiation from cell phones and computers, drink more water, and resolve an emotional trauma that preceded the onset of depression and fatigue.

I teach my clients how to be "health detectives" by applying the **UCP** to their own health issues. Understanding this paradigm, and applying the principles and solutions in this book to your health issues, is the first step in taking personal responsibility for your health.

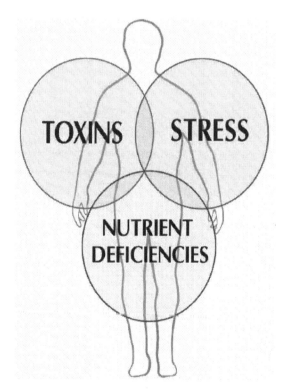

Image by Crystal Castle Graphics

Chapter 3

Nutrient Deficiencies

"Today, more than 95% of all chronic disease is caused by food choice, toxic food ingredients, nutritional deficiencies and lack of physical exercise."

- *Mike Adams, Author, Investigative Journalist, Educator*

I remember one of my mentors once told me that almost everyone is in a state of sub-optimal health, because they are deficient in optimal levels of key nutrients including fatty acids, vitamins, minerals, enzymes, bioflavonoids and antioxidants. A three-year study, surveying the dietary habits of over 16,000 Americans, found that a large portion of the population **consistently fails to meet even the minimal intakes** recommended in the Dietary Reference Intake (DRI) for many key nutrients. The study published in the Journal of Nutrition (August 2011) concluded: "Without enrichment and/or fortification and supplementation, many Americans did not achieve the recommended micronutrient intake levels set forth in the Dietary Reference Intake."

The National Health and Nutrition Examination Survey (NHANES) 2003-2006 reviewed the average intake of 19 essential micro-nutrients in 16,110 people including key vitamins such as vitamins A and K and important minerals such as calcium and magnesium. The only positive news (if you can call it that) from the study was that the majority of the American population showed a sufficient minimum intake of the following nutrients: vitamin B-6, folate, zinc, thiamin, riboflavin, niacin, vitamin B-12, phosphorus, iron, copper and selenium. The study notes that fortified food and/or taking supplements (food with synthetic nutrients added to it) are the reasons the majority of these daily requirements are met. In other words, conventional food is clearly deficient in key nutrients and must be fortified to prevent nutrient deficiency based disease.

On the down side of the study, a large percentage of the population showed intakes of other key nutrients that are clearly below the minimum daily requirements. These nutrients are magnesium, calcium and vitamins A, C, D and E.

- 25% do not get enough vitamin C
- 34% do not get enough vitamin A
- 38% do not get enough Calcium
- 45% do not get enough Magnesium
- 60% do not get enough vitamin E
- 70% do not get enough vitamin D

It is important to note that the minimum daily requirement for a nutrient is usually defined as the lowest amount that can be taken in order to not develop a "deficiency" and an associated disease or health condition. For example, the minimum daily requirement for vitamin C is 90 mg. If you take less than this amount for an extended period of time, you will develop scurvy. Although taking 90 mg will keep scurvy at bay, it is not the amount needed for optimal health. In fact, chronic sub-optimal vitamin C levels will eventually contribute to many health problems, including a suppressed immune system and cardiovascular disease. These daily requirements were never designed with "optimal health" in mind; they were designed to minimize the risk of disease. However, health is much more than just the absence of disease.

The major reasons people develop nutrient deficiencies are the following:

- The produce we eat is grown in nutrient depleted soil and the animals we eat are raised on nutrient depleted feed.

- The produce we eat is often not fully ripened when picked and thus the food does not reach maximum nutrient content. This is a practice used to minimize transport and storage spoilage.
- Irradiation. As more food is irradiated to ostensibly reduce risk of pathogens on food, those foods subjected to irradiation are depleted of key nutrients such as vitamins A, C, E, B-2, B-3, B-6, B-12 and K, thiamine and folic acid.
- Nutrient loss due to overcooking. It turns out that the traditional rules about heat, water, time and nutrient loss are all true. The longer a food is exposed to heat, the greater the nutrient loss. Being submersed in hot water (boiling) creates more nutrient loss than steaming (surrounding with steam rather than water) if all other factors are equal.
- We use up more nutrients including B vitamins, vitamin C, vitamin E, antioxidants and important minerals, such as calcium and magnesium, to cope with and neutralize free radicals from increased stress and exposure to toxins.
- With increased incidence of chronic digestive issues such as constipation, indigestion, candida and parasite infections, people absorb less of the nutrients from their already nutrient depleted foods.

Decline in Nutrient Content of Food

A landmark study on the nutrient content of the nation's food supply by Donald Davis and his team of researchers from the University of Texas, Department of Chemistry and Biochemistry, was published in December 2004 in the Journal of the American College of Nutrition. They studied U.S. Department of Agriculture nutritional data from both 1950 and 1999 for 43 different vegetables and fruits, and found "reliable declines" in the amount of protein, calcium, phosphorus, iron, riboflavin (vitamin B-2) and vitamin C over the past half century. Davis and his colleagues attributed this declining nutritional content in food to the preponderance of agricultural practices designed to improve traits (size, growth rate, pest resistance) rather than nutrition.

The Organic Consumers Association cites several other studies with similar findings: A Kushi Institute analysis of nutrient data from 1975 to 1997 found that average calcium levels in 12 fresh vegetables dropped 27%; iron levels 37%; vitamin A levels 21% and vitamin C levels 30%. A similar study of British nutrient data from 1930 to 1980, published in the British Food Journal, found that in 20 vegetables the average calcium content had declined 19%; iron 22%; and potassium 14%. **Yet another study concluded that one would have to eat eight oranges today to derive the same amount of vitamin A as our grandparents would have gotten from one.**

The likelihood that you are suffering from one or more key nutrient deficiencies is almost certain if you eat a diet of non-organic food, and you do not supplement your diet with a high quality vitamin/mineral supplement. For those who eat a primarily organic diet, you are still likely to have sub-optimal levels of key nutrients and suffer from sub-clinical nutrient deficiencies.

Here are four steps to maximize your chances of your body having all the nutrients it needs to function optimally:

1. Eat a healthy, organic diet that provides a foundation for your nutritional needs including optimal macro nutrient (protein, fat, carbohydrate) ratios.
2. Take a whole food based multivitamin-mineral formula to provide insurance for any key micro-nutrient deficiencies you are likely to have, even if you eat an organic diet.
3. Use self-assessment of symptoms or basic lab tests to determine any specific micronutrient (vitamins, minerals, antioxidants) deficiencies you may have after taking a high quality food-based multivitamin/mineral supplement. (See Resource Guide for testing options).

4. Support healthy digestion by taking a high quality probiotic supplement and use herbs and digestive enzymes to support your digestion when needed.

Our bodies are made out of protein, fats, minerals and water. All of your organs and glands (including your brain) need energy from food including key micronutrients such as vitamins, enzymes and trace minerals in order to function optimally.

The first step to prevent nutrient deficiencies is to have high quality sources of food. Specifically, this should include organic vegetables and fruits, organic raw nuts and seeds and organically fed and naturally raised (free-range) animal protein sources, such as eggs, meat and poultry, free of antibiotics and hormones and wild-caught fish from clean waters.

A complete, balanced meal is composed of the following three macronutrients:

PROTEIN: meat, fish, fowl, eggs, organic raw cheese, nuts, seeds, beans, legumes.

CARBOHYDRATES: organic vegetables, fruits, whole grains, beans and legumes.

FATS: butter, olive oil, coconut oil, fatty animal proteins, raw nuts and seeds, raw nut butters, avocados and olives.

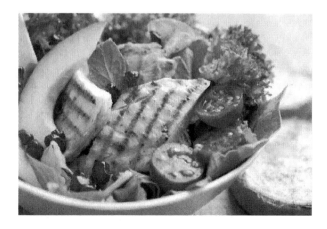

To optimize energy, mood balance and mental clarity it is important to balance these macronutrients in each meal. If you eat a reasonably balanced diet of protein rich foods, organic fruits and vegetables and healthy fats such as butter, olive oil, fatty meats, raw nuts and seeds – it is virtually impossible to have macro-nutrient (protein, carbohydrate, fat) deficiencies. Most of our nutrient deficiencies will be in the micronutrient categories of vitamins, minerals, enzymes, antioxidants and other phytonutrients.

Fundamental Principles of Diet and Nutrition

The following **six dietary principles** are the foundation for optimizing your health through nutrition:

1. Pay attention to how your mind and body feel with different ratios of proteins, fats and carbohydrates. Some people need more protein and fats; others need more carbohydrates. Your body is unique and only by paying attention to what works for you will you find the right diet.

> *Use the **Daily Diet Diary** (See Forms Section) to track how you feel using key indicators such as energy, mood and mental clarity. Make adjustments according to how you feel with both the types of foods you eat and with macronutrient ratios in accordance with either your intuition or your metabolic type. Note: For more information on Metabolic Typing see William Wolcott's book in my Resource Guide.*

2. Eat whole (unprocessed) organic food as much as possible including fresh organic fruits and vegetables, raw nuts and seeds, and organically fed and naturally raised grass fed beef and bison, free-range poultry and eggs and wild caught fish. Organic food is more nutrient dense and has less toxicity than commercially raised foods. Experiment with eating anywhere from 1/3 – 1/2 of your food raw and/or sprouted. Eat more salads, fresh vegetable juices, raw nuts and seeds and bean and seed sprouts.

3. Cook animal protein slowly at 225 degrees Fahrenheit or less to reduce oxidative damage to protein and fats. Since your cells are made out of amino acids and fatty acids, the quality of these building blocks will determine the quality and function of your cells. Cooking at above 225 degrees Fahrenheit will damage the molecular bonds in proteins and fats and therefore will have a cumulative negative impact on cell function.

4. Reduce sweets, caffeine and alcohol. Each of these have a depleting effect on nutrient reserves and/or hydration levels.

5. Make sure you digest your food properly. Chew your food thoroughly; take digestive enzymes with cooked foods if you have poor digestion and use herbal teas such as peppermint, ginger and fennel to help digestion. If protein digestion is poor, use Betaine hydrochloride (food based hydrochloric acid) to support digestion. Eat high quality cultured foods such as yogurt, kefir and sauerkraut or take a high quality pro-biotic on a regular basis. The key to health is digesting your food efficiently and absorbing nutrients needed for fueling and repairing your body.

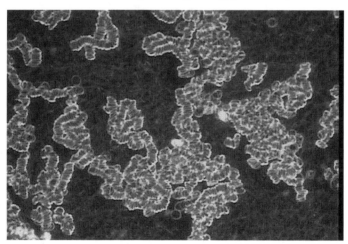

Excess sugars and carbohydrates as well as poor protein digestion will contribute to red blood cells sticking together as seen above. The net result of blood like this will be reduced oxygenation and poor circulation leading to fatigue and increased chronic pain.

6. Allow your digestive system to rest periodically. Eat your larger meal at lunchtime, eat a lighter dinner and avoid eating after 8 pm. Also, take periodic mini-fasts every 2-3 days by skipping a meal or two and drinking extra water or fresh juices in place of a meal. This is the key principle of *intermittent fasting*.

Some of the documented benefits of **intermittent fasting** include:

- reduces inflammation and free radical damage
- increases levels of nerve growth factors (NGF) which extends life of brain neurons and has been shown to improve memory and learning
- increases human growth hormone in both men and women
- regulates blood sugar levels by normalizing insulin and leptin sensitivity
- lowers triglyceride levels

Intermittent fasting is not a diet, but rather a dieting pattern. In simpler terms, it's making a conscious decision to skip certain meals. By fasting and then feasting on purpose, intermittent fasting means eating your calories during a specific window of the day, and choosing not to eat food during the rest.

Here are two ways to take advantage of intermittent fasting:

- Regularly eat during a specific time period. For example, only eating from noon-8 PM, essentially skipping breakfast. Some people only eat in a 6-hour window, or even a 4-hour window.

> - Skip two meals one day, taking a full 24-hours off from eating. For example, eating on a normal schedule (finishing dinner at 8 PM) and then not eating again until 8 PM the following day. This pattern is most easily incorporated into your eating program by doing it every 3rd or 4th day.

For more information on intermittent fasting see Addendum A, *The Handbook of Intermittent Fasting*

Remember that food is composed of protein, carbohydrates, fats, vitamins, minerals, enzymes, and an array of phytonutrients and water. It is critical that your body gets all the nutrients it needs to function properly or your health will suffer. Your body must get adequate protein and fats to function properly and can use fats for sources of energy. High carbohydrate foods (including grains) are not necessary for your body to function and for some people can have a damaging impact on brain, cardiovascular and overall health. (Note: Read *Grain Brain* by David Perlmutter, MD for a more in depth exploration of the adverse effects of grains and high carbohydrate foods on health.)

The importance of fresh air and sunlight

Before discussing specific nutrient deficiencies, let's talk about even more fundamental deficiencies, which are often overlooked, namely fresh air and sunlight. Oxygen is essential for life and fresh air on a regular basis is necessary for vibrant health. A rule of thumb is to get fresh air at least every 4 to 6 hours during your waking hours. In other words, if you're working in an office building, factory, warehouse or any other indoor facility for a full eight hour shift, try to take your lunch break outdoors or open your office window if possible. The next best option is to put oxygen giving plants and an air purifier in your home and/or office to optimize your lung's access to fresh air.

Sunlight is often overlooked as a nutrient we need for health; however, the sun not only helps your body make vitamin D (which is necessary for a healthy immune system and building strong bones) but it also regulates your hormones and sleep cycles.

It is critical for optimal health to address any nutrient deficiencies that your diet alone doesn't cover.

To assess nutrient deficiencies, there are lab tests including blood tests and hair tissue mineral analysis, which are available through healthcare professionals. You can also assess deficiencies based on your symptoms, many of which I will review in the section on common nutrient deficiencies. As a general rule, I recommend everyone use a food-based vitamin-mineral supplement to minimize the risk of developing a key nutrient deficiency. The vast majority of nutrient deficiencies will be micro-nutrient deficiencies such as vitamins, minerals and phytonutrients which can be easily addressed with an organic diet and high-quality, easy to assimilate supplements.

> *Phytonutrients are plant compounds other than vitamins and minerals and include:*
>
> ▲ *enzymes*
>
> ▲ *antioxidants*
>
> ▲ *polyphenols such as bioflavonoids, flavonols and pycnogenols.*

Food based supplements integrate nutrients, such as vitamins, minerals, enzymes, antioxidants and polyphenols, into a food base for easier assimilation. These supplements usually have lower doses of the vitamins and minerals, are easier to assimilate and are less likely to create nutrient imbalances or toxicities than isolated nutrient supplements. (See the Resource Guide supplement section for my top recommendations for this important supplement category.)

Organic food vs. non-organically grown food

Hippocrates, the father of medicine, said, *"Let your food be your medicine and your medicine be your food."*

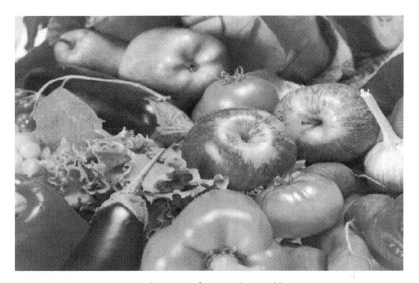

Fresh organic fruits and vegetables

Non-organically grown produce sprayed with pesticides, herbicides and grown with chemical fertilizers have numerous disadvantages over organically grown foods including:

- Pesticides, insecticides, herbicides and fungicides actually block a plant's ability to manufacture antioxidants and polyphenols. Without these key nutrients, plants are handicapped and too weak to fight off pests. These key nutrients protect your cells from toxins, decrease inflammation and reduce your risk of allergies and degenerative diseases like arthritis, heart disease and cancer.

- Bio-accumulation of pesticides increases the risk of many health problems including: allergies, chronic fatigue, headaches, suppressed immune and endocrine function and more.

- Children and fetuses are most vulnerable to pesticide exposure due to their less-developed immune systems and because their bodies and brains are still developing. Exposure at an early age can cause developmental delays, behavioral disorders and motor dysfunction.

- Pregnant women are more vulnerable due to the added stress pesticides put on their already taxed organs. Plus pesticides can be passed from mother to child in the womb, as well as through breast milk. Some exposures can cause delayed effects on the nervous system, even years after the initial exposure.

- Recent studies reveal that organic foods, especially raw or non-processed, are also substantially more nutritious than foods sprayed with pesticides and herbicides. They contain higher levels of beta carotene, vitamin C, D and E, polyphenols, cancer-fighting antioxidants, flavonoids that help ward off heart disease, essential fatty acids and essential minerals. (See Resource Guide for Organic Consumers article on nutrient comparison between organic vs. non-organic food.)

Organic food is more nutritious and less toxic than non-organic food and should be prioritized in your diet.

The Importance of Vitamins and Minerals

> *"You can trace every sickness, every disease and every ailment to a mineral deficiency"*
>
> — Linus Pauling, two-time Nobel Prize Winner

Vitamins

While vitamins are not sources of energy themselves nor are they significant building materials of the body, they are essential as co-enzymes in the regulation of metabolic processes. Vitamins serve as protection against toxins and are catalysts in the production of energy. In other words, deficiencies of crucial vitamins will compromise your body's ability to function optimally.

Vitamins are essential for life and generally cannot be synthesized by the body. We must obtain them from our diet or from nutritional supplements. A chronic deficiency of any vitamin will eventually have an adverse effect on your health.

Minerals

There are 103 known minerals; at least 18 of these are necessary for good health. Minerals are essential constituents of all cells and body fluids. Mineral imbalance is epidemic. Osteoporosis is on the rise in our nation; 30 million people in the U.S. over fifty are susceptible to fractures caused by mineral deficiencies in their bones. Close to 1/3 of the women in America will be diagnosed with osteoporosis in their lifetime. Zinc deficiency is becoming more common, evidenced by such health issues as prostate cancer, breast cancer, hormonal imbalances, hydrochloric acid deficiency, and skin cancer. Magnesium is involved in at least 300 functions in the body. Magnesium can be depleted by stress and diets high in sugar, caffeine or alcohol. A large percentage of my clients are magnesium deficient.

Some of the roles minerals play in the body include:

- Acting as co-factors for enzyme reactions. Enzymes will not function without minerals. All cells require enzymes to work and function.
- Maintaining acid-base balance within the body.
- Facilitating the transfer of nutrients across cell membranes.
- Supporting nerve transmission.
- Helping to contract and relax muscles.
- Helping to regulate our body's tissue growth, fluid regulation and cellular osmosis.
- Providing structural and functional support for the body.

> Check Addendum B for a list of vitamins and minerals, including how they function in your body and their food sources.

It is very difficult to get all the vitamins and minerals your body needs to function optimally from food alone, even if that food is organically grown.

In 2002, I experimented with taking no nutritional supplements and only used whole organic foods for my nutritional needs. I ate organic fruits and vegetables and drank on average two fresh organic green vegetable juices per day. I ate only the highest quality organic, grass-fed beef and free-range poultry. The milk I drank was fresh, unpasteurized milk from grass-fed cows from Amish Farms. The eggs were free-range and the freshest I had ever eaten.

After about a year on this superb diet, I began to develop a few minor health problems including a chronic intestinal candida overgrowth and feeling more fatigued. I ran a hair tissue mineral analysis and found that I was deficient in many minerals including calcium, magnesium, copper and zinc.

My plan of action to improve my health and to reverse these new symptoms included an herbal cleansing program for the candida overgrowth, a high quality pro-biotic, an adrenal support formula and a high quality whole-food multivitamin/mineral formula at moderately high doses for a few months. Within three months my health issues were resolved and upon retesting my hair sample, I found that my mineral levels were all in the excellent range again. This experience taught me that eating organic food does NOT necessarily mean that I will receive all the nutrients I need for optimal health. If there are not adequate minerals in the soil in which the food is grown, these nutrients will not be in the food you eat. Organic food, although more nutrient-dense than non-organic food, may not have all the nutrients you need.

Common Nutrient Deficiencies

In this section I will discuss some of the most common nutrient deficiencies, the symptoms you may experience from the deficiencies and the best food and supplement sources for these nutrients.

WATER

While some do not consider water a nutrient, try living without it for a few days. The bottom line is your body is made up of over 70% water and the quality and quantity of this water has a direct impact on every aspect of your health.

Dehydration – the lack of water – is a very common deficiency. A life changing book I highly recommend on the subject of the importance of water for your health is, *Your Body's Many Cries for Water: You Are Not Sick, You Are Thirsty!* by F. Batmanghelidj, MD (See Resource Guide Addendum A.).

Symptoms of dehydration include: fatigue, headaches, muscle cramps, dark urine, chronic pain.

The primary cause of dehydration is insufficient intake of water on a daily basis. For optimizing metabolic cellular function, your water consumption should be calculated by taking your body weight in pounds, divide by two and drink that many ounces of water per day. For example, if you weigh 150 pounds, you would need to drink 75 ounces of pure water per day. Preferably, this would be in 4 ounce increments every 30 minutes since the body can only absorb about 4 ounces every half hour.

Another contributing factor to dehydration is the excess consumption of diuretics such as sugar, tea, coffee, sodas, alcohol and many medications. For every dehydrating beverage drink an extra 8 ounces of water and for every 30 minutes of exercise drink an extra 4 ounces on top of your baseline water intake.

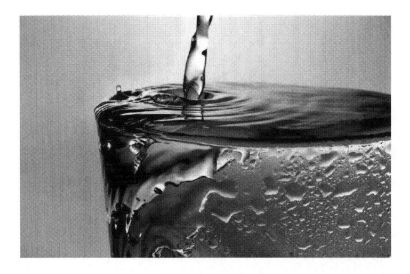

The best sources of water are thoroughly filtered tap water or clean spring water and fresh vegetable juices. Other than coconut water, most concentrated fruit juice is too high in sugar to consume on a regular basis for optimal health. (See the Resource Guide section on health-related products for high quality water filtration systems.)

ENZYMES

> *"Eighty percent of our body's energy is expended by the digestive process... Because our entire system functions through enzymatic action, we must supplement our enzymes. Aging deprives us of our ability to produce necessary enzymes.. The medical profession tells us that all disease is due to a lack or imbalance of enzymes. Our very lives are dependent upon them!"*
>
> – Dr. DicQie Fuller, author of The Healing Power of Enzymes

Although enzymes are also commonly overlooked in the discussion of nutrient deficiencies, these essential nutrients are critical for health. Enzymes are made in your body and can be consumed from foods and supplements. Enzymes are heat sensitive and begin to be destroyed by heat at around 115 Fahrenheit.

Enzymes are proteins that catalyze metabolic functions in the body. Your body synthesizes thousands of enzymes. Enzymes are required for your body to function properly, because without enzymes you wouldn't be able to breathe, swallow, drink, eat or digest your food. To do all of these things, your body needs some help. You must have enzymes to help perform these tasks. In short, enzymes are an absolute necessity for life.

Enzymes literally are your body's work force. They are responsible for constructing, synthesizing, carrying, dispensing, delivering and eliminating the many ingredients and chemicals our body uses in its daily business of living. There are an endless array of symptoms created by enzyme deficiencies including: fatigue; poor digestion and constipation; reduced vitality and stamina; slower rate of recovery from exercise, injury or illness; poor memory; suppressed immune function and increased susceptibility to infections; sluggish liver function and decreased capacity to remove toxins from your body and many more.

The primary causes of enzyme depletion are: low intake of raw, sprouted and cultured foods, chronic stress, overcooking of food and high levels of exposures to toxins. The best sources of enzymes are found in raw and sprouted foods such as: raw fruits and vegetables; bean, nut, seed and grain sprouts; superfoods like bee pollen, spirulina and chlorella; raw honey and raw protein foods such as sushi and raw eggs. Digestive and systemic enzyme supplements are also great sources of enzymes to support our enzyme levels and prevent enzyme depletion.

Although there are dozens of enzymes our body requires, I listed enzymes as a general category for nutrient deficiencies. Most people who eat a diet of primarily cooked food and do not use enzyme supplementation will likely benefit from the full spectrum of enzymes. These are found in a high quality enzyme supplement, such as the ones listed in the Resource Guide and by eating more raw, sprouted and cultured foods. (See Resource Guide supplement section for enzymes supplements.)

> *I have used enzyme therapy extensively for my own healing and in my practice. One year I had a man in his early 80s come to see me with an occluded carotid artery. The blockage was diagnosed by a medical doctor with an MRI and was in the 90% range. I put my client on a good diet and two supplements: a high quality whole food based vitamin C to help repair the artery and 3 capsules 2 x day of a systemic enzyme formula taken on an empty stomach to clear up the blockage in the artery. Several months later he had a second MRI and found that the blockage had reduced to less than 20%.*

MAGNESIUM

"Every known illness is associated with a magnesium deficiency...magnesium is the most critical mineral required for electrical stability of every cell in the body. A magnesium deficiency may be responsible for more diseases than any other nutrient."

— *Dr. Norman Shealy*

Magnesium deficiency is the most common nutrient deficiency I see in my practice and is very easy to correct with proper supplementation. The first symptoms of deficiency can be subtle. As most magnesium is stored in the tissues, leg cramps, foot pain or muscle 'twitches' can be the first sign. Other early signs of deficiency include loss of appetite, nausea, vomiting, fatigue and weakness. As magnesium deficiency worsens, numbness, tingling, seizures, personality changes, abnormal heart rhythms and coronary spasms can occur.

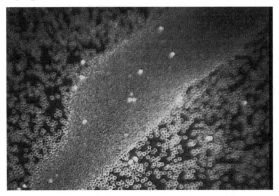

Red blood cell aggregations as seen in this picture are caused by either magnesium deficiency or dehydration.

Symptoms involving impaired contraction of smooth muscles include constipation, urinary spasms, menstrual cramps and difficulty swallowing. Your central nervous system can also be markedly affected. Symptoms include insomnia, anxiety, hyperactivity and restlessness with constant movement, panic attacks, agoraphobia and premenstrual irritability. Magnesium deficiency symptoms involving the peripheral nervous system include numbness and tingling. Symptoms or signs of the cardiovascular system include palpitations, heart arrhythmias and angina due to spasms of the coronary arteries, high blood pressure and mitral valve prolapse.

The causes of magnesium deficiency include: low magnesium levels in the soil or a diet low in magnesium-rich foods, high calcium intake and high levels of acidic waste and toxins, which deplete the plasma and tissue levels of magnesium. Vegetables are generally high in magnesium while animal products are generally low in magnesium.

Sources of magnesium include green leafy vegetables, nuts, seeds, dark chocolate and halibut. This is the most commonly supplemented nutrient I recommend for my clients. A typical dosage is between 400-800 mg per day. You may need more if you're very toxic or have a long-standing deficiency.

Some of the significant health improvements of addressing a magnesium deficiency include: elimination of chronic muscle cramps/spasms, better sleep quality, alleviation of constipation and ending of irregular heartbeat (arrhythmia).

IODINE

Symptoms of iodine deficiency include: fatigue, dry skin, hair loss and low libido. All signs of hypothyroidism are due to an iodine deficiency. In fact, it is impossible to have healthy thyroid function if you are iodine deficient. Recent national surveys have shown that 11% of Americans are iodine deficient and this number is probably much higher considering the extremely low levels needed to meet FDA recommended dosage.

Causes include removal of iodized salt, lack of iodine in soil, insufficient intake of iodine rich foods in diet, excess consumption of goitrogenic rich foods such as: soy products, peanuts, uncooked vegetables such as cauliflower, broccoli, Brussels sprouts. The displacement of iodine is caused by chlorine and fluoride, which are found in municipal water supplies, mouthwash and toothpaste. In addition, bromines, commonly used in refined flour products and other processed foods, also displace iodine. (See Resource Guide, *Overcoming Thyroid Disorders.*)

Iodine has four important functions in your body:

- Stabilization of metabolism and body weight
- Brain development in children

- Fertility
- Optimization of your immune system (iodine is a potent anti-bacterial, anti-parasitic, anti-viral and anti-cancer agent)

Sources of iodine include seafood, seaweed (kelp, dulse, hijiki) and free-range egg yolks. Three of the best iodine supplements are: Prolamine iodine, Lugol's, Iodoral. (See Resource Guide.)

Recommended Dosage: RDA is 150 mcg. Japanese eat up to 12.5 mg per day from food sources.

To test for iodine deficiency, see Resource Guide under Testing: www.doctorsdata.com.

VITAMIN K

Symptoms of vitamin K deficiency include osteoporosis, tartar buildup, arterial calcification and even heart disease. Vitamin K is essential for calcium deposition into bones. Without vitamin K, calcium can build up in arteries. Causes include a lack of vitamin K in diet if commercially raised meats are consumed.

Sources of vitamin K include free-range egg yolks, aged cheese, goose liver, fish eggs, miso soup and other fermented soy products. Good supplement sources of vitamin K include high quality vitamin butter oil and K2 liquid from several companies, including Thorne Research.

VITAMIN B-12

Symptoms of vitamin B-12 deficiency include hair loss, anxiety and depression, anemia, Alzheimer's, incontinence, low blood pressure, shakiness.

Causes include poor digestion and absorption of nutrients from animal products, low hydrochloric acid levels and gut flora imbalances. One key cause is simply underestimating the amount we need.

Sources of vitamin B-12 include red meat, liver, sardines and salmon. Regarding supplementing with B-12, I recommend sublingual vitamin B-12 for easier absorption and assimilation.

Recommended Dosage: If you're a meat eater, have good digestion and occasionally eat liver you'll be fine. If not, take 1 mg per day of sublingual methylcobalamin (cobalt bound vitamin B12).

VITAMIN D

Symptoms of vitamin D deficiency include: Seasonal Affect Disorder, depression, osteoporosis and susceptibility to colds and flu and overall suppressed immune function.

Causes include lack of exposure to sunlight, not consuming enough foods high in vitamin D and often a lack of knowledge that you may need to take a vitamin supplement and underestimating the amount you need.

Sources: The best source of vitamin D precursor hormone is sunlight. Next best sources would be wild caught salmon, tuna, flounder and free-range eggs.

Recommended Dosage: 800 IU day and up. I try to get 2,000 IU per day or get it from sunlight. Between 5 and 30 minutes of sun exposure to your unprotected face, arms, legs or back between the hours of 10 am and 3 pm two to three times every week is enough for your body to produce all the D3 it needs. The darker your skin the closer to 30 minutes you'll need.

Vitamin D (D3 specifically) is an oil soluble steroid hormone that is formed when your skin is exposed to ultraviolet B (UVB) radiation. However, the vitamin D that is formed on the surface of your skin does not immediately penetrate into your bloodstream. This is called pre-vitamin D. Pre-vitamin D is synthesized in your skin and makes a home in the oil glands. From there, it goes into your bloodstream. If you shower before the pre-vitamin D has been absorbed and converted to vitamin D, it will wash off and your vitamin D levels will not rise. (NOTE: Sunscreens are toxic and not only do nothing to prevent skin cancer, but have been linked to increased skin cancer incidents. The best approach to block ultraviolet rays is to use a natural antioxidant cream.)

So how long should you wait before bathing? Evidence shows it takes up to 48 hours before you absorb the majority of the pre-vitamin D that was generated by exposing your skin to the sun! That is TWO DAYS for those of you doing the math! Crazy right? Who can wait that long? Simply bathe or shower with water and use a natural soap only in areas where you feel you must wash.

Note: In climates where exposure to sunlight in the winter months is reduced, it is essential to take a vitamin D supplement.

ZINC

Zinc deficiency symptoms include lack of appetite, moodiness, reduced sense of taste and/or smell, a weaker immune system and susceptibility to colds and flu.

The primary causes of a zinc deficiency are depleted soil sources and copper toxicity. Strict vegetarian diets are notoriously low in zinc and high in copper, which causes poor digestion and lack of absorption of this vital nutrient.

The best sources of zinc include liver, pumpkin seeds, beef, raw milk and cheese, oysters, beans, green peas, crimini mushrooms, spinach and sea vegetables.

Recommended Dosage: is 15 mg per day.

Zinc is a critical nutrient for men's hormonal balance and optimum testosterone levels.

POTASSIUM

Symptoms of potassium deficiency include muscle cramps, body weakness, fatigue, anorexia, low blood pressure, constipation and depression.

Causes include excess sodium in the diet, excess exercise and/or sweating, adrenal fatigue or burnout in addition to the use of many medications, including diuretics and some asthma medications, magnesium deficiency and a poor diet.

Reliable sources of potassium include bananas, avocados, sweet potatoes, beets, artichokes, most fruits and vegetables, yogurt, kidney beans and almonds.

Recommended Dosage: for adults is 4,700 milligrams of potassium a day.

About 1/3 of my clients have low tissue levels of potassium. This is often related to chronic stress and low functioning thyroid and adrenal glands. Nutritional support, detoxification and reducing chronic sources of stress are the way to get potassium levels to normal.

Summary

If you make sure you have a healthy diet centered around high quality proteins such as meat, poultry, fish and eggs cooked at low temperatures, organic fruits and vegetables and high quality fats such as butter, olive oil, coconut oil and raw nuts and seeds, you will have taken the first step toward vibrant health and disease prevention. Next you will want to supplement that excellent diet with a whole food-based multivitamin-mineral formula. Finally, you will want to assess (either through testing or symptoms) any nutrient deficiency, which may be contributing to your health issues.

It is also very important to note that it is possible to take too much of an isolated vitamin or mineral. You will be less likely to create a toxic accumulation of a mineral or fat soluble vitamin, if you supplement your diet with a whole-food based formula as I recommend.

Nutrient Deficiencies

Not only are nutrients literally the building blocks of every cell in our body and necessary for all metabolic functions of the body, they are also the key vitamins, minerals, amino acids and antioxidants, which we need to protect ourselves from environmental toxins such as chemicals, heavy metals and radiation.

Now that we have addressed the importance of nutrition, let's talk about how toxicity impacts your health.

Chapter 4

Toxicity

"Darwin's theory of natural selection still applies, but there have been some changes. The fittest are now those who detoxify the most efficiently."

-David Vaughan, clinical nutritionist and detoxification expert.

Most people overlook toxins as a factor in the quality of their health, primarily because toxins are invisible to the naked eye. Conventional medicine and all our major institutions including government agencies, higher education, religions and many businesses (such as pharmaceutical, processed food and chemical industries) either downplay or disregard the impact of toxins on our health, unless lethal or near lethal doses are taken.

What is a toxin?

A toxin is any substance that creates irritating or harmful effects, undermines our health or stresses our biochemistry or organ function.

Toxins harm our health in two ways:

1. Toxins damage cells and the organs, tissues, glands and systems that create those cells. When these organs, tissues or glands are damaged their functional capacity diminishes. For example, chemicals can damage blood vessels, which scar and over time can lead to blockages in the blood vessels. Toxins lead to degenerative diseases and increase your risk of both chronic and acute health problems.

2. Your body uses vital nutrients to process and eliminate toxins. These same nutrients are necessary for fueling and regenerating your body. So when your exposure to toxins increases, if you do not increase your nutritional intake, your body will feel more tired, function less optimally and degenerate faster.

> *Your rate of detoxification must exceed your intake of toxins or you will age faster, develop chronic illnesses and die prematurely. This basic maxim must be understood if you are serious about taking charge of your health.*

To maximize your rate of detoxification you must optimize the following:

- **Hydration** – water helps both flush toxins out and transport nutrients into cells.
- **Elimination** – efficient bowel function and optimization of the other detoxification pathways such as kidneys, lungs and skin.
- **Digestion** – what is not digested becomes toxic to your body. The process by which food is converted into amino acids, fatty acids, glucose, vitamins and minerals that can be absorbed and assimilated by the body is accomplished in the digestive system by the mechanical and enzymatic breakdown of foods into simpler chemical compounds.
- **Assimilation** – the uptake of nutrients into cells and tissues and consequent building up into more complex substances (as opposed to breaking down for the release of energy, which is respiration). Proper hydration and blood circulation impact nutrient assimilation as well as the presence of nutrient co-factors. For example, vitamin D levels must be adequate for calcium to be assimilated into bone. Nutrient balance is therefore a necessary prerequisite for proper assimilation.

- **Sleep** – getting your eight hours of sleep per night is not only essential to function optimally during the day but it has also been found to be the critical element necessary for toxin removal from the brain. A 2013 study conducted by the University of Rochester Medical Center, which was published in the journal, *Science*, reveals that the brain's unique method of waste removal – dubbed the glymphatic system – is highly active during sleep, clearing away toxins responsible for Alzheimer's disease and other neurological disorders. Furthermore, the researchers found that during sleep the brain's cells reduce in size, allowing waste to be removed more effectively.

Detoxification is a normal body process of eliminating or neutralizing toxins through the colon, liver, kidneys, lungs, lymph glands and skin.

With approximately 70% of your body composed of water, the condition of that water is critical for the functioning of your body. Your body fluids – blood, plasma, interstitial fluids (fluid between cells) – are a lot like seawater and have high concentrations of sodium chloride. In addition to sodium and chloride other electrolytes (mineral salts) in your body include: potassium, calcium, magnesium, bicarbonate, phosphate and sulfate. Without the proper balance of water and electrolytes, toxic metals and chemicals can interrupt proper cell function.

Some of the well-documented effects of toxins on the body include:

- Toxic metals such as aluminum, mercury, lead and cadmium damage the brain, nervous system, digestive and endocrine systems, liver, kidneys and cardiovascular system.

- Volatile Organic Compounds (VOCs) such as acetone, benzene, ethylene glycol, formaldehyde, methylene chloride, perchloroethylene and toluene are known to cause both short term adverse health effects on breathing and respiration as well as long term damage to liver, kidneys and the central nervous system.
- Bisphenol (BPA) is a synthetic compound used in plastic bottles. BPA is an estrogen-mimicking chemical, which contributes to lowered testosterone and fertility levels in both men and women. It has also been linked to increased incidence of breast cancer in women.

Much of mainstream culture and corporate enterprise is dependent upon toxic foods, toxic forms of energy (fossil fuels and nuclear) as well as toxic medical treatments. It can be difficult to confront the impact of environmental toxins on the world, let alone your own personal health, because it invites us to alter our world-view. Despite the overwhelming task of dealing with this reality, we must face the facts and take action to protect ourselves, and the environment. There is really no difference between how we are treating our planet and how we are treating our bodies.

Understanding the nature and extent of the toxic load we are carrying is an essential step in taking responsibility for your health. The three primary categories of toxins that we are exposed to are:

- **chemicals**
- **heavy metals**
- **radiation**

The compounding negative effect of these toxicities equate to your toxic load. This load is influenced not only by the cumulative effect of multiple exposures to a vast variety of chemicals, heavy metals and radiation, but also by:

- duration of exposure – longer is worse
- quantity of exposure – more is worse
- strength and vitality of your organs which support detoxification, e.g. liver, lungs, kidneys and bowel. This vitality is a product of nutritional status, overall stress levels and genetics.

CHEMICALS

Over the past 60 years there have been over 80,000 chemicals introduced into the environment. There has been virtually no safety testing for the effect of these chemicals on human beings and none on the compounding negative effect of these chemicals with each other and other forms of toxins such as heavy metals and radiation.

Chemicals are toxic byproducts of our modern industrial age. They are capable of damaging the proteins and fatty acids, which make up our cells, our hormones and the very DNA which encodes our body's every function. Chemicals also deplete the body of vital nutrients we need to produce energy and heal.

Chemicals damage:

- **our immune system causing infections, allergies and cancer;**
- **our endocrine system causing thyroid and adrenal disease and diabetes;**
- **our nervous system causing learning and behavior problems;**
- **our reproductive system causing dysfunction in sexual health and fertility levels.**

Toxicity

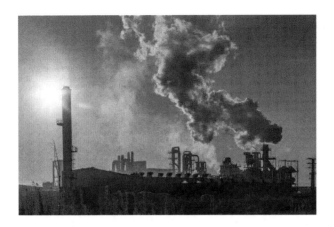

Did you know that:

- refined sugar (which is a synthetic compound, i.e. chemical) suppresses your immune system, is a primary contributing factor to cardiovascular disease and is one of the primary causes of ADD?
- the chemical used in dry cleaning (perchloroethylene) damages the nervous system?
- common pesticides used on commercially grown produce (non-organic) can suppress the immune system and impair normal hormone function?

Toxic chemicals include the following categories:

Chemical Solvents (VOCs): perchloroethylene (dry cleaning/neurotoxin), trichloroethylene, glycol ethers, turpentine and more. Also found in degreasers, adhesives, fuels, polishes, coolants, detergents, etc. These toxins poison the nervous system, liver, glands and more.

Food Additives called excitotoxins, which include: MSG, aspartame, NutraSweet, sulfites, hydrolyzed protein and more. These goodies poison the brain and nervous system and contribute to ADD, ADHD, poor memory, Alzheimer's and many more health problems.

Synthetic xenoestrogens are widely used industrial compounds, such as PCBs, BPA, phthalates and pesticides. These compounds mimic estrogen in the body and contribute to **reduced testosterone and sperm counts,** increase of body fat, premature aging, prostate swelling and prostate cancer.

> *Pthalates are chemicals used to soften industrial plastics. Pthalates disrupt hormone function and are correlated to reproductive and developmental health disorders. They are found in numerous petroleum based products including: PVC (polyvinyl chloride), Vinyl flooring, lubricants, oils, weather stripping, pool covers, children's toys, food wrappers and plastics cosmetics, nail polish and makeup, detergents, plastic water bottles and plastic bags.*

Pharmaceutical drugs – side effects are so numerous as to often take up paragraphs in minute print for any one particular drug. These side effects include everything from liver damage, skin outbreaks, digestive disorders, mood imbalances, allergies, anaphylactic shock, coma and death.

Benzenes are a carcinogenic class of chemicals which are found in many commonly used products including: cigarette smoke, vehicle emissions, building materials, plastic bottles, styrofoam, glues and adhesives, liquid detergents, solvents, textured carpets, and paint removers. Benzenes cause anemia, suppression of the immune system and are strongly associated with bone and blood cancers such as leukemia.

Remember these categories of chemicals are layered on top of our ever-present exposure to common chemicals which are very difficult to completely avoid such as:

- **pesticides, herbicides, insecticides**
- **chlorine and fluoride – found in municipal water supplies**
- **hair dyes and nail polish**

- **polybrominated diphenyl ethers (BPDE) used in flame retardants found in new cars, children's sleepwear and numerous other commercial and industrial products perfluorooctanoic acid (PFOAs) is part of a larger class of chemicals known as perfluorinated compounds (PFCs). PFCs and PFOA in particular, are the bases for non-stick coatings on cookware; stain guards on clothing, upholstery and carpet; and waterproof clothing.**

As you can see it is virtually impossible to avoid exposure to these chemicals. It is important to remember that although our bodies have mechanisms to remove these chemicals, it takes energy and nutrients to mobilize and support these forces. The more exposures to chemicals one has, the more energy and nutrition one will need to clear them from your body.

As if this tsunami of chemicals were not enough to deal with, agribusiness and geneticists have come up with yet another bizarre "food product" to foist upon an unwitting public.

Genetically Modified Organisms (GMOs) are in an infamous class of their own.

Unlike hybrid seeds, GMO seeds are not created using natural, low-tech methods. GMO seed varieties are created in a lab using high-tech and sophisticated techniques like gene-splicing.

Furthermore, unlike hybrids, which cross-pollinate different but related plants, GMOs often cross different biological kingdoms, such as a bacterial strain with a plant.

For example, Monsanto has crossed genetic material from a bacteria known as Bt (*Bacillus thuringiensis*) with corn. The goal was to create a pest-resistant plant. This means that any pests attempting to eat the corn plant will die since the pesticide is part of every cell of the plant. Imagine the cumulative damage done to your intestines, liver and nervous system and every cell in your body by eating a diet of GMO foods.

The resultant GMO plant, known as *Bt Corn*, is itself **registered as a pesticide with the EPA** along with other GMO Bt crops. In other words, if you feed this corn to your cattle, your chickens, or yourself, you'll be feeding them and yourself an actual pesticide — not just a tiny pesticide residue. In essence, Monsanto and other GMO producers are creating foods which are both legally and literally poison.

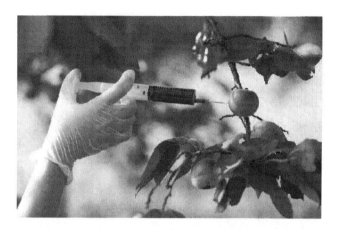

Here are ten easy ways to protect against exposure and accumulation of toxic chemicals:

1. **Eat organic food** as much as possible including naturally raised, free range, hormone free meats, poultry and eggs.

2. **Avoid food additives** such as NutraSweet, Aspartame, MSG and GMO foods.

3. **Replace chemical based body care products with organic, plant based, non-chemical products.** (See The Green Beauty Guide: Your Essential Resource to Organic and Natural Skin Care, Hair Care, Makeup, and Fragrances in resource section).

4. **Be conscious of your environment and avoid or reduce exposure to chemicals** (cleaners, solvents, paint, pesticides, plastics, etc.) Once you condition yourself to use natural products for everything from cleaning products and lawn care to cooking and drinking containers, you will gradually reduce your overall toxic load and your health will improve.

5. **The amino acid complex glutathione is both a potent antioxidant and is involved in detoxification.** It binds to fat-soluble toxins, such as heavy metals, solvents, and pesticides, and transforms them into a water-soluble form that can be excreted in urine. Boost glutathione levels with foods and supplements including: low-temperature processed whey protein, cottage cheese, eggs, meat, fish, poultry, garlic, onions, milk thistle, N Acetyl Cysteine, L-Glutamine, L- Glycine and Alpha Lipoic Acid.

6. **Consume foods or a supplement high in the organic compound Indole 3 Carbinol found** in cruciferous vegetables such as broccoli, cauliflower, brussels sprouts and kale. Indole 3 Carbinol rich foods help detoxify xenoestrogens and also serve as potent antioxidants with anti-carcinogenic properties.

7. **Drink sufficient amount of pure water.** Take your body weight in pounds and divide by two, drink between two-thirds and 100% of that number (for example, if you weigh 160 pounds that would be between 60-80 ounces per day) in ounces of pure water from glass or stainless steel containers per day. Please, NO PLASTICS!

8. **Increase consumption of organic fruits and vegetables high in pectin fibers**, which bind with chemicals and heavy metals in the gut and facilitate safe removal from your body. Best sources include: apples,

citrus fruit (include the white inner part of peel), bananas, grapes, carrots, beets and cabbage. Also consider a pectin supplement such as Chem Detox by Premier Research Labs (See Resource Guide Nutritional Supplement section).

9. **Sweat regularly.** Sweating through exercise and saunas helps to remove chemicals and heavy metals. Aerobic exercise will also move toxins through the lymph system. If you use a steam sauna make sure that the water used has filtered out chemicals such as chlorine and fluoride.

Two studies published in 2012 found that sweating enhances the elimination of dangerous endocrine-disrupting petrochemicals.

The first study, published in the Journal of Environmental Health, involving 20 subjects made to undergo induced sweating, found that the ubiquitous petrochemical **Bisphenol A** (BPA) was excreted through sweat, **even in some individuals with no BPA detected in their serum or urine samples.** This clearly indicates that the body uses sweat to rid itself of the BPA that has bio-accumulated in tissue.

The second study by the same research group (this time published in Scientific World Journal) found that phthalate, a plasticizer tied to breast cancer and various other conditions associated with endocrine disruption, was present in concentrations twice as high in their sweat compared to their urine. In several individuals phthalate was found in the sweat but not in their blood serum, "...suggesting the possibility of phthalate retention and bio-accumulation."

---

10. **Only use pharmaceutical drugs if you have no other non-toxic option to regulate your health.** Consult a doctor trained in both conventional and alternative medicine.

Since 1997, I have repeatedly seen myriad chemicals in human blood with a dark-field microscope. These chemicals appear as bright blue, green, yellow, red, orange or whitish crystals and clear up when the exposure to chemicals is reduced and/or the body's capacity to filter toxins from the bloodstream is improved. Sometimes, if a person activates cellular detoxification, more toxins will appear in the blood until the detoxification pathways are properly supported and the body is more efficient at clearing the accumulated toxic load. It is important to prepare the body with the correct balance of nutrients and support strategies before activating deep cellular detoxification. Not doing so will not only minimize the effectiveness of your detoxification program, but can actually cause damage to the body. (See image of live blood below.)

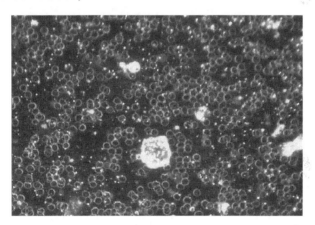

This is what a blood stream full of chemicals and other toxins looks like under a dark-field microscope. The small round circles are red blood cells, the larger white forms are white blood cells and the bluish crystals are toxins. This person's liver was overwhelmed with toxins, he felt exhausted, nervous and had pain throughout his body.

The blood pictured in the above image can be cleared up with the following two steps:

1. Reduce or stop exposure or ingestion of the offending chemicals whether it be household cleaning products, chemical additives, paint fumes or hair dye, etc.

2. Utilize simple detoxification support strategies such as increasing water intake, sweating in a sauna and taking a liver cleansing herbal formula.

Within several days or weeks (depending on the severity of the toxic load) the blood picture will be significantly improved and you will feel much better.

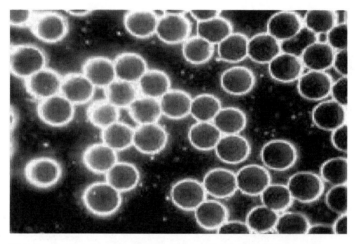

This is what healthy blood looks like under a dark-field microscope at 50 x red blood cells are round, have smooth membranes and the background is free of chemicals and other toxins.

Your bloodstream is like a river. It transports oxygen, nutrients and other life-giving agents throughout your body to maintain health. It is also a highway for detoxification, delivering cellular waste to the liver and kidneys for elimination from the body. The state of your blood can serve as a predictor of health and provide an indication of illness well before symptoms appear.

Unlike the thousands of chemicals we are exposed to, there are only two dozen or so toxic metals we come across in our life times; however, these dozen or so heavy metals can be even more devastating to our health than the chemicals I listed above.

HEAVY METALS

> *"Most organic substances are degradable by natural processes. However, no metal is degradable...they are here to stay for a long time."*
>
> Dr. Henry Schroeder, MD, world authority on trace elements.

Heavy metals (HMs) are mineral elements such as mercury, lead, arsenic, cadmium, aluminum, nickel, beryllium, antimony, bismuth, barium and radioactive elements such as uranium, radium, strontium, etc. They are called "heavy metals" because they have a higher number of atomic particles per atom than lighter elements (such as carbon, oxygen, hydrogen, nitrogen), so they weigh more and thus are difficult to remove from your body's cells than lighter elements like most chemicals. They usually don't occur in living organisms or organic molecules. HMs are typically locked up in rocks or in earth and therefore are not commonly present in air, water or food.

Also, note that minerals needed in lesser quantities are usually toxic in greater amounts. Examples are copper, iron, manganese, selenium and vanadium. Even calcium and sodium can be quite toxic in excess.

So, how do we get heavy metals into our bodies?

HMs are released into the environment due to modern industrial mining and refining and in the heating and melting of mineral ore for use in the manufacturing and chemical industries. They are also released into the atmosphere due to the burning of coal, trash and petroleum products. Air pollution carries HMs into our food supply such as dairy, fish, meat and vegetables. They are also used in common medicines such as vaccines and antibiotics and in dental fillings and crowns.

How do heavy metals impact our health?

Toxic metals replace nutrient minerals in enzyme binding sites. When this occurs, the metals inhibit, over stimulate or otherwise alter thousands of enzymes. An affected enzyme may operate at 5% of normal activity. This may contribute to many health conditions. Toxic metals may also replace other substances in other tissue structures. These tissues such as the arteries, joints, bones and muscles, are weakened by the replacement process.

Toxic metals may also simply deposit in many sites, causing local irritation and other toxic effects. They also fuel intestinal fungal, candida and parasite infections that are difficult or impossible to eradicate until the toxic metal cause is removed.

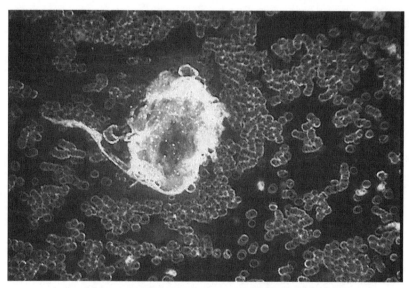

A large protoplast seen in the center of this dark-field blood picture indicating leaky gut.

One way fungal and candida infections impact our health is to throw off one's gut flora balance which leads to what is known as intestinal permeability or "leaky gut syndrome". This can be seen in live blood as the large waste particle seen in the above blood picture. These bowel toxins recirculate and often get deposited in tissues causing inflammation, pain and irritation to the immune and nervous system.

The following are the most common heavy metals I have seen in my practice including their sources and health problems they cause.

MERCURY

> "Mercury is the most toxic and poisonous non-radioactive, heavy metal substance on the planet,"
>
> -Tom McGuire, DDS, author of <u>Tooth Fitness:</u> <u>Our Guide to Healthy Teeth</u>

Mercury is now number three on the Top 20 list of toxic substances compiled by the U.S. Agency for Toxic Substance and Disease Registry. Only lead and arsenic rank higher. The most common source of mercury toxicity is from dental amalgam fillings and metal dental appliances.

In 1989, the EPA declared that amalgams are a hazardous substance under the Superfund Law. Ironically, this law established that **outside** of your mouth mercury amalgams must be stored in unbreakable, tightly sealed containers away from heat and cannot be touched. However, both the EPA and the American Dental Association consider mercury that is stored **inside** your mouth in the form of dental fillings as non-toxic.

For additional numerous articles and studies on mercury amalgam toxicity, please check out Savvy Patients at www.savvypatients.com.

Mercury and other heavy metals, destroy important proteins in the body; many of them enzymes, hormones or cell receptors.

Mercury can be found in three forms: elemental, inorganic and organic. All forms are highly toxic.

Elemental mercury is found in liquid form. It can easily vaporize at room temperature and can penetrate the human Central Nervous System (CNS).

Sources of elemental mercury include: barometers, batteries, calibration instruments, dental amalgams, electroplating, fluorescent and mercury lamps, jewelry, paints, silver and gold production, semiconductor cells and thermometers.

Inorganic mercury is mostly found in mercuric salt form (e.g. batteries) and is highly toxic. It gains access to the body orally or through the skin and accumulates in the kidneys.

Sources of inorganic mercury include: cosmetics, disinfectants, explosives, embalming fluid, ink manufacturing, perfume, photography, tattooing inks, vinyl chloride production and wood preservation.

Organic mercury is absorbed more completely from the GI tract than inorganic mercury and is distributed uniformly throughout the body accumulating in the brain, kidneys, liver, hair and skin.

Sources of organic mercury include: antiseptics, antibacterial, fungicides, germicides, insecticides, laundry products, paper manufacturing, wood preservatives and thimerosal, a preservative used in vaccines and antibiotics.

According to a study done on 1,300 patients by the Foundation For Toxic Free Dentistry (FTTD), symptoms of mercury toxicity fall into the following categories:

Neurological impact includes chronic or frequent headaches; numbness and tingling; dizziness; ringing or noises in the ear; tremors in hands, feet, lips, eyelids, tongue; lowering of pain threshold.

Psychological disorders related to mercury in the body include irritability, nervousness, shyness or timidity, loss of memory, inability to concentrate, mental confusion, mood changes, lack of interest in life/hobbies, ADD or ADHD, decline of intellect, loss of self confidence, anger and loss of self-control, depression, crying spells, anxiety, drowsiness and insomnia.

Oral Cavity problems including: bleeding gums, bone loss and loosening of teeth, foul breath, excessive salivation, metallic taste, white patches on the gums or mouth, ulcerations, burning in the mouth or throat, and black tissue pigmentation.

Gastrointestinal complaints include symptoms such as: bloating and excessive gas, abdominal cramps, constipation or diarrhea, irritable bowel syndrome, colitis, nausea, loss of appetite, voracious appetite and obesity and excessive thirst.

Cardiovascular problems such as: irregular heartbeat, feeble and irregular pulse and alterations in blood pressure and arterial plaque.

Mercury toxicity can also include inflammatory and immunological problems such as: chronic fatigue syndrome, fibromyalgia, rheumatoid arthritis, allergies, sinusitis, asthma, muscle weakness and joint pain.

Other problems can include excessive perspiration without fever; low body temperature (sometimes with clamminess); skin rashes especially around the face, head and neck; dim or double vision and hypoxia (lack of oxygen).

According to statistics compiled by FTTD on 1,569 patients from 6 different reports an average of 81% of the symptoms were cured or improved after amalgam removal.

Case of Laura

Laura, age 32, presented with severe digestion problems. Bloating, gas, constipation, candida overgrowth, allergies and sensitivities to foods. She could not eat a single piece of fruit without having a candida flare up. She could only afford to remove one dental amalgam every two months. After 18 months

> she was mercury amalgam free and her candida overgrowth was gone, she could eat a sweet treat once in a while with no adverse reaction. In addition to removing her dental amalgams she used a food based supplement to assist in the detoxification of heavy metals and a high quality pro-biotic supplement to help re-establish healthy flora levels in her GI tract.

LEAD

Major **sources of lead toxicity** include: air pollution, exploding ammunition, auto exhaust, batteries, contaminated soils, cosmetics, fertilizers, hair dyes, insecticides, lead-based paint, pesticides, water run through lead pipes and tobacco smoke.

Lead poisoning symptoms can be vague and often go undiagnosed including: Abdominal pain, ADD, adrenal insufficiency, allergies, anemia, headaches, hyperactivity, fatigue, impotence, numbness, vertigo, etc. Lead in food is a primary health concern. Food produced close to heavy traffic or lead emitting industries, lead-soldered food cans and fertilizers with sewage sludge added to them will all increase lead levels in foods. Another surprising source of lead toxicity is the drinking from lead glazed tea and coffee mugs.

> I had high levels of lead in 2002 and found out that the tea mugs I had been drinking from were the source of my lead toxicity. Go to www.mugrevolution.com to order a lead free mug.

To reduce lead in foods eat fresh foods and be sure to wash and peel all non-organic root vegetables.

ALUMINUM

Major **sources of aluminum toxicity** include: aluminum foil, aluminum canned food and beverages, antacids, aspirin, dust, auto exhaust, treated water, vanilla powder, nasal spray, milk products, table salt, tobacco smoke, antiperspirants, bleached flour, ceramics and commercial cheese.

Aluminum toxicity symptoms and conditions include: flatulence, headaches, dry skin, weak and aching muscles, senility, liver and kidney dysfunction, neuro-muscular disorders, anemia, Alzheimer's disease, ALS (Lou Gehrig's disease), memory loss, hemolysis, leukocytosis, Parkinson's disease, constipation and more.

Recent studies indicate that **aluminum toxicity is a significant contributor to neurological disorders** such as Alzheimer's disease, Parkinson's disease, senility, dementia and various other neurological disorders.

Aluminum toxicity is cumulative and therefore the health hazard to the elderly is significantly greater.

CADMIUM

Major sources of cadmium toxicity include: air pollution, batteries, ceramic glazes/enamels, cigarette smoke (first and second-hand), tap and well water, food (if grown in cadmium contaminated soil), paints, fungicides, mining sites, and seafood.

Symptoms of cadmium toxicity include alopecia (hair loss), anemia, arthritis, hypertension, infertility, kidney disease, cardiovascular disease, migraine headaches, neurological damage, damages the immune system and diabetes.

Cadmium damages the cell membranes and allows for increased permeability of the cells leading to the storage of heavy metals into the cells. One cigarette contains 16-24 mcg of cadmium of which the body absorbs 50%.

> The danger of toxic metals is greatly aggravated today by the low mineral content of most of our food supply. An abundance of vital minerals protects against toxic metals. Vital minerals

> compete with toxic metals for absorption and utilization in enzymes and other tissue structures. The first line of defense against toxic metal accumulation is making sure you have no mineral deficiencies.

Top seven steps to take to reduce HM exposure and detoxify heavy metals:

1. **Have your mercury amalgams removed.** These poisons have a powerful negative impact on your brain, nervous system, digestion and immune system. Make sure you use a dentist who is properly trained in the safe removal of mercury dental amalgams. (See www.iaomt.org for a list of mercury-free dentists.)

2. **Avoid obvious heavy metal sources in environment:** aluminum canned beverages, canned tuna, pesticide laden food, aluminum laced antiperspirants, copper IUDs, non-essential medications, unnecessary vaccinations, lead glazed coffee and tea mugs, cigarette smoke, both first and second-hand.

3. **Do a heavy metal detoxification program at least once a year.** See Detoxification Program in Addendum D.

4. **Eat foods and use herbs that are beneficial for detoxifying heavy metals including:** cilantro, chlorella (a single cell algae) coconut oil, beet root and greens, dandelion greens, milk thistle and medicinal mushrooms such as shiitake, reishi and maitake.

5. **Sweat regularly – exercise and saunas.** Both chemicals and heavy metals are removed in perspiration.

Toxicity

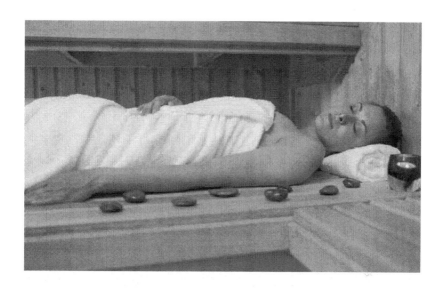

A groundbreaking 2011 study published in the Archives of Environmental and Contamination Toxicology found: "Toxic elements were found to differing degrees in each of blood, urine, and sweat. Serum levels for most metals and metalloids were comparable with those found in other studies in the scientific literature. **Many toxic elements appeared to be preferentially excreted through sweat.** Presumably stored in tissues, some toxic elements readily identified in the perspiration of some participants were not found in their serum.

Induced sweating appears *to be a potential method for elimination of many toxic elements from the human body*. The researchers also made the important observation that, "Bio-monitoring for toxic elements **through blood and/or urine testing may underestimate the total body burden of such toxicants.** Sweat analysis should be considered as an additional method for monitoring bio-accumulation of toxic elements in humans."

6. **Make sure you have sufficient levels of minerals** since these nutrients are your first line of defense against heavy metal toxins accumulating in your cells. Use a whole-food vitamin-mineral supplement, eat seaweed from clean waters and drink fresh organic vegetable juices including wheat-grass juice. These are mineral dense foods which will help block your cell receptor sites from attracting heavy metals. If a Hair Tissue Mineral Analysis indicates a deficiency in a key mineral it is necessary to supplement that mineral until levels are sufficient to protect your cells from heavy metal toxicity.

7. **Take bentonite, montmorillonite, french green clay or pyrophyllite clay baths** to support detoxification of heavy metals. These clays draw out and attract chemicals and heavy metals through your skin pores. (See Resource Guide for clay products).

Testing for heavy metals can be done in three ways:

Urine testing – this is done with what is called a "chelation challenge" in which heavy metal levels are tested in the urine prior to administering a chelation agent such as DMPS or DMSA. This test measures both heavy metals and minerals and is accurate. The downside is that it is expensive, has to be done by a physician and many people feel sick when mobilizing stored levels of toxic metals.

Blood test – Can test both minerals and heavy metals. Must be done by a physician, can be expensive. Tests for recent exposures to heavy metals but can not determine if metals have been stored in organs, glands and other tissues.

Hair Tissue Mineral Analysis (HTMA) – Tests for tissue levels of minerals and heavy metals, does NOT have to be done by a physician, is less expensive than the other tests and has no side effects. (See Resource Guide for labs.)

RADIATION

> *"Independent research findings, including our own, show that cell phones damage the DNA of brain cells and sperm in animal models. Research lavishly funded by industry to counteract the results from the independent science should be taken with caution."*
>
> -Narendra P. Singh, Research Associate Professor, Department of Bioengineering, University of Washington (Seattle)

Up until the late 1990s, chemicals and heavy metals were the two primary sources of toxicity in our lives. During a blood cell analysis microscope training in 1999, one of my mentors, Michael Coyle, told me that radiation (specifically non-ionizing radiation) will be the number one environmental factor affecting our health in the 21st Century.

There are two types of radiation: ionizing and non-ionizing. We all know that radioactive waste and nuclear bombs (i.e. ionizing radiation) are very dangerous and we have strict regulations protecting us from these exposures. Many of us don't realize that the less dangerous non-ionizing radiation (which includes cell phones, cordless phones, microwaves, cell phone towers, smart meters, computers and electrical appliances) can have a larger adverse impact on our health because this form of radiation is not only not regulated it is commercially advocated at every turn.

Ionizing:

This type of radiation is powerful enough to damage DNA and break molecular bonds: x-rays, gamma rays, nuclear bombs, radioactive waste products of nuclear reactors like uranium and cesium are examples of ionizing radiation. It is highly regulated and universally accepted as dangerous to our health at certain levels of exposure. Symptoms of low-level exposure can be as mild as headaches, fatigue, nausea, and at high levels organ destruction, cancer and death.

Non-ionizing:

This type of radiation is less powerful, not well regulated and includes electromagnetic radiation produced by electric current, radio waves, microwave ovens, radar stations, television (cathode ray tube), video display terminals (VDT's), computers, high voltage lines, infrared and fluorescent lights and sunlamps (i.e. tanning booths which emit ultraviolet light).

Symptoms of excess exposure to non-ionizing radiation include: fatigue, headaches, reduced cognitive function including memory, foggy thinking, depression, sleep disturbances, hormone imbalances, ADD, ADHD, increased risk of certain types of cancers (brain cancer) for high volume cell phone usage.

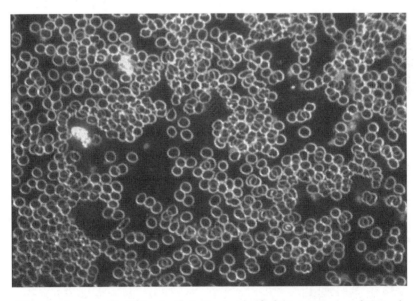

The membranes of red blood cells in the top half of this picture are damaged by electromagnetic radiation as demonstrated by the bizarre shapes.

> **Case of Vince:** I had a client who came to me with overwhelming chronic fatigue and after working with him for 8 months or so he was feeling great. I helped him eat a more nutritious diet, provided nutritional support for his liver and adrenal glands to work more efficiently and improved his digestion and circulation. Things were improving and he came back to my office to have his blood rechecked. When I looked at his blood, I saw many of his red blood cells were misshapen and damaged. He was complaining of being tired again and was puzzled. I began questioning him about changes he had made and he couldn't think of any.
>
> His blood looked like he had a big dose of either x-rays or some other form of radiation. Still, we couldn't figure out what was causing his blood cells to be so damaged. Finally, I asked him if he was using a computer or laptop more often. He said that, in fact, he had just bought a laptop and had been watching a Netflix movie almost every night for the past two weeks, and had kept his laptop on his lap during the movie. Bingo, that was it! I told him to either watch the movies on a desktop or keep the laptop away from his body at least a foot. Within 2-3 months his blood started to look better and his energy returned.

Here are six simple steps to protect yourself from low levels of ionizing radiation, and moderate to high levels of non-ionizing forms of radiation:

1. **Use one level tablespoon of thyme to one pint of boiling water and steep for twenty minutes.** After cooling and straining it, drink two cups a day. The tea also works toward cleansing and building the blood lymphatics and the thyroid and thymus, in addition to assisting in the elimination of radiation poisoning.

2. **Add kelp, dulse and other seaweeds in your daily diet.** One-half tsp. of purple dulse flakes per day is sufficient iodine for your thyroid to function well.

3. **Use radiation detox clay baths.** There are several good clay products on the market these days. One of the best is made by LL Magnetic Clay's *radiation detox clay* bath. 1-2 baths per week is all that is needed. (See www.magneticclay.com)

4. **Test your home and office for high levels of electromagnetic radiation.** Get a Trifield meter (which measures magnetic, electric and radio wave fields) from www.lessemf.com. If you have high levels where you sleep and/or work use their shielding technologies. Call the number on the website. These people know their stuff.

5. **Reduce or eliminate your use of wireless products and when using your cell phone use either the speaker function or an air tube headset.** I highly recommend reading, *Cell Phones: Invisible Hazards in the Wireless Age: An Insider's Alarming Discoveries* by Dr. George Carlo. (See Resource Guide.)

6. **Use a comprehensive detoxification/antioxidant formula** to reduce bio-accumulation of chemicals, metals and radiation and to protect your cells from being damaged by these environmental toxins. **D-Toxol** by Ultra Life and Dr. Drucker's **All in One** formula are two excellent choices. (See Resource Guide supplement section.)

By now you may feel overwhelmed by this information. However, I have good news. Understanding about nutrient deficiencies and toxins and implementing some of the suggestions I've made will start a transformation in your health as soon as you put into practice the recommendations in this book.

I have taught thousands of people how to reduce their toxic load and significantly improve their health with these **four easy steps:**

1. **Evaluate your toxic load** by taking a toxicity survey and if necessary doing lab tests for more specific toxicity assessment. (See Forms and Surveys #2.)

2. **Strengthen your nutritional shield** to these toxins by implementing the suggestions in Chapter 2 including eating a healthy, organic diet, supplementing your diet with potent super foods such as wheat-grass juice, bee pollen and chlorella; and taking a high quality whole food vitamin-mineral supplement.
3. **Reduce or avoid exposure** to sources of chemical, heavy metal and radiation toxicities.
4. **Do a seasonal or bi-annual detoxification program** as outlined in Addendum D.

Chapter 5

Stress

"The secret of health for both mind and body is not to mourn for the past, not to worry about the future, or not to anticipate troubles, but to live in the present moment wisely and earnestly."

– Buddha

Although most of my work with clients focuses on nutrient deficiencies and toxicities, there are often cases where the primary impediment to vibrant health is some form of stress. Physiological, emotional and mental stress are major factors impacting our health. My mentor, Michael Coyle, used to tell me that given decent nutrition and a relatively moderate level of toxicity, emotional factors are the most important issues affecting our health.

Our mind, beliefs and emotions (psyche) play a huge role in our overall health. The beliefs and emotions we carry directly affect our biochemistry, nervous system and immune system and indirectly affect every cell, tissue, organ and other body system. The mind-body connection in health is very well established in many areas including: immunity, digestive function, blood pressure and cardiovascular health. When someone is depressed, discouraged or feeling hopeless, there is quantifiable drop in immune function. Even low level anxiety and fear can impair both digestive and cardiovascular health. Chronic anger can increase our blood pressure and the risk of cardiovascular disease.

From a biological perspective stress makes perfect sense. If you are about to be attacked by a lion, your stress response could save your life. Unfortunately, the same stress response is also triggered by chronic worrying. So when we worry about money, health, work and relationship issues, these worries appear to our body as a threat to our survival and kick in the "fight or flight" hormone response.

To make matters worse, unlike most other animals in which the stress response rapidly dissipates, once the threat is removed, humans have great difficulty turning off the stress response. Our worries and fears literally bathe our cells with stress hormones like cortisol and epinephrine making our heart beat faster and muscles tighten.

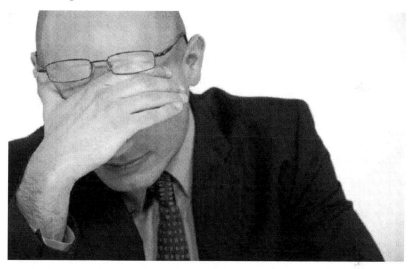

The Japanese word "Karoshi" literally translates as death by over work or stress. Like the Japanese, we live in a culture that puts a premium on financial success and accomplishment. Little attention is given to living in balance with life and its natural rhythms.

How does stress actually impact our body?

When we are under stress, our adrenal glands produce excess cortisol, which diverts energy away from other more essential functions. Under chronic stress we experience the following biological effects:

- Immune system suppression
- Reduced capacity to regulate inflammatory response
- Reduced capacity to digest our food
- Increased bowel permeability and thus waste flooding into the bloodstream
- Increased oxidative damage to cells including DNA damage and reduced telomere length

> At the ends of the chromosomes are stretches of DNA called **telomeres**, which protect our genetic data and make it possible for cells to divide. Telomeres have been compared with the plastic tips on shoelaces because they prevent chromosome ends from fraying and sticking to each other, which can scramble an organism's genetic information, and could lead to diseases such as cancer.

High cortisol levels are linked to the following chronic health conditions:

- Diabetes
- Heart disease
- Obesity
- Depression
- Gastrointestinal disorders
- Infertility

Studies on animals have shown that increased stress levels:

- Clog arteries – reducing blood flow to the heart
- Reduce brain cell size and have a negative impact on learning and memory

Fortunately, cortisol levels are neutralized by the hormone oxytocin known as the "cuddle hormone". Oxytocin increases when we have positive social interaction, care for others and experience nurturing touch. In fact, oxytocin is released in the stress response inviting us to connect with others. Oxytocin has been shown to increase regeneration of heart cells.

We experience stress at three levels:

- Physical
- Emotional
- Mental

Physical symptoms of stress include low energy, insomnia and loss of sex drive, aches and pains, muscle tension, poor digestion, lowered immunity, headaches and chest pain.

Emotional symptoms include frustration, being easily agitated and feeling overwhelmed, feeling bad about oneself and avoiding social contact.

Mental or cognitive symptoms include constant worrying, racing thoughts, forgetfulness, pessimism, poor judgment and an inability to focus.

Understanding what is causing chronic stress in your life, and addressing these factors effectively, is essential to your well being.

My Stress Story: I became very disillusioned with the legal system early in my career. On top of this I had a very difficult time connecting with women during this period of my life and my parent's divorce a few years earlier had hit me hard. I lost faith in God, spirituality, our political system, the family, the legal system and finally myself. I experienced a perfect storm of emotional factors, which contributed to the collapse of my

> health. I responded to these stresses by drinking more alcohol and sinking deeper into depression.
>
> It took seven years to work through enough of these stresses and develop healthier responses to life's disappointments before my health would recover. I know that even with all the detoxification and nutritional support I did for my health, I would not have restored my health completely if I had not cleared up the sources of stress and transformed my cynical view of life.

Over the course of a ten-year period, in addition to all my nutrition and detoxification programs and practices, my healing journey included the following:

- Meditation
- Chanting and sound healing
- Network Chiropractic – a type of body centered emotional healing modality
- Reading uplifting spiritual books
- Spending more time with children and family
- Completing a course focused on forgiveness
- Letting go of my career as a lawyer and trusting I would find a new one that better suited me
- Moving to a place where I felt free to be myself
- Connecting with more like-minded people

Adopting A Wellness Mindset

The best way to deal with stress is to adopt a wellness mindset. A wellness mindset is one that makes your happiness and well being a top priority. Many of us live according to society's rules and expectations. We often live for work or for taking care of others to our detriment.

Here are my top recommendations for adopting a wellness mindset:

1. Acknowledge the aspects of your health that are working for you.

Start by making an inventory of all the ways your body and mind work well. For example, can you walk without pain? Can you hear and see well? Do you have to think in order to digest your food and breathe air? Many of us tend to take for granted how well our bodies are functioning for us most of the time.

Constantly focusing on our problems can create low level anxiety and even depression. You can cultivate more of a wellness mindset by acknowledging how your body is working well on many different levels. This exercise brings to your awareness how your body is perfectly designed to heal and regenerate itself.

2. Make sure you're getting adequate nutritional support during stressful periods, including:

- B complex vitamins
- Adaptogen herbs such as Siberian ginseng, American ginseng, astragalus, ashwagandha, suma and licorice.
- Cortisol reducing formulas such as Laminine. (See Resource Guide supplement section, www.supportforyourbody.com)
- Adrenal support formulas, which will have adrenal glandulars or protomorphogen extracts along with B vitamins and vitamin C among others. The best of these formulas is *Drenamin* made by Standard Process. See Resource Guide on supplements.

3. Take breaks.

Make your happiness and well being a top priority. This includes short breaks during the day to get away from work by taking a walk or just lying down for a short rest. Get up from your desk every 30-60 minutes to stretch. I also recommend taking at least a short three-day getaway once a month and a longer 1-2 week break every few months and ideally a long vacation once a year.

> My blood never looked more healthy than after a two week vacation in the Caribbean. During my vacation my diet was not ideal, yet my blood cells were in perfect shape, my immune system was very strong and the blood was clear of any noticeable toxicity. Even when my life is too busy to take longer vacations, I have found shorter breaks from work have greatly reduced my stress. It is important to leave behind all work and as much responsibility as possible during these breaks.

4. Do what you enjoy.

There's nothing better for relieving stress than being able to do something that gives you a lot of pleasure and satisfaction and makes you feel good about yourself.

5. Spend time in nature including implementing *Earthing* practices.

Our bodies are designed to be in nature. Modern life insulates us from our natural habitat and connection to nature. Just as getting sunlight is crucial for our endocrine system, immune system, circadian rhythms and overall health, so is making direct physical contact with the earth itself. *Earthing* is a practice in which you make direct skin contact with the earth on a regular basis in order to absorb earth energies. **Being barefoot on the grass for 20-30 minutes per day is the easiest way to implement *earthing* into your daily life.**

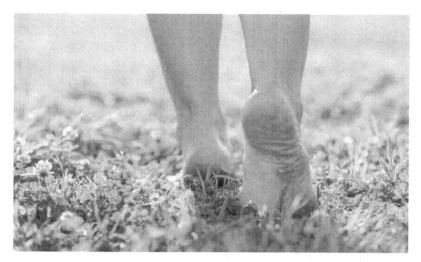

The principle of earthing is based on an electron transfer from a larger organic body to a smaller one. Since the earth is much larger than you and me, we absorb massive amounts of healing electron energy when we have direct skin to earth contact. I highly recommend reading *Earthing* (See Recommended Reading in Addendum A), which goes into great detail on the science behind this healing phenomenon.

6. Connect to Source.

> "There are no atheists in foxholes."
>
> – Author unknown

This quote refers to the human impulse to turn to a higher source when under extreme stress and fear. Why wait for high levels of stress or illness to drive you toward a higher source? Our connection to higher source is always here waiting for us to ask for help. The book I've highly recommended on this topic is *The Power of Now* by Eckhart Tolle.

When I felt alone in the world with only my rational mind to navigate health, career and personal issues, I often felt overwhelmed. When reason and will power were exhausted and I opened up to what I called "Truth and God" my life changed.

I remember saying early in my illness that I was willing to do anything to improve my health, as long as I didn't have to believe in God. I was very down on any spiritual teaching and was committed to being cynical. Gradually, however, I began studying books on the merging of science and spirituality. I also had some very unique and unexpected metaphysical experiences. Slowly, I opened up to the benevolent forces of the universe and the possibility of life beyond this dimension.

7. Increase positive social interaction and touch.

Oxytocin "the cuddle" hormone is released when we have good connections with people we love and feel nurturing toward or nurtured by another. Oxytocin neutralizes excess cortisol levels. Humans need touch and love in order to feel integrated and whole. Intimacy does not have to be sexual to be healing. Receiving a massage, getting and giving regular hugs, in addition to honest communication and heart-felt connections, are all essential for emotional and physical health. Paradoxically, stress triggers the pituitary gland to release oxytocin, which primes a person to reach out, connect to others and alleviate the adverse effects of stress. If we trust our response to stress, we can actually improve our health.

When we experience stress, we have a choice. We can either close down, turn to drinking, drugs or medications, or we can choose to connect to family, friends and turn to Spirit. Stress can actually be the catalyst for you to grow and experience more connection and meaning in life.

The Importance of Letting Go of the Past

Another way we experience stress is by holding on to negative experiences from the past. Many of us have had traumatic or disappointing experiences, which color our view of life and limit us from reaching our full potential. For example, pain from past experiences can impair our ability to not only experience life fully, but also to be fully healthy. Unresolved issues related to important areas of life including: intimate relationships, parents, children, career, health traumas and more can cause contractions in our mind and body. This contraction is felt as a weight that can reduce our energy, vitality and overall health.

Fortunately, there are tools to help us clear and release these contractions and allow us to move forward. One of my favorite tools for facilitating the release of unresolved trauma and stress is **The Completion Process**. I want to thank and acknowledge Bill Lamond, author of the book, *Born to Lead*, for being the source of this valuable tool. This process supports clearing unhealthy beliefs and emotional charge so that one can move ahead with greater freedom in important areas of one's life. I've used this process to resolve issues in my relationships with women and family members in addition to issues related to my career and my health.

The Completion Process has three objectives:

1. To acknowledge what has served you well in whatever area of life you are completing.
2. To release any painful or negative experience you have in relationship to what you are completing.
3. To both forgive and thank the important people who are connected to this area of your life.

First, establish what aspect of your past you would like to complete.

Here are some common examples:

- Your last or current job
- Your last or current relationship with a partner
- Your relationship to your parents

- An illness you experienced
- A business relationship that went sour
- Your relationship with the opposite gender
- Your relationship to money
- Where you live

Here is an example of **The Completion Process** relating to one's last intimate relationship. Ask yourself the following five questions and write in a journal your complete answer to each question:

1. Regarding my first marriage, what was pleasurable, profitable or beneficial to me?
2. Regarding my first marriage, what was painful or caused me suffering?
3. Regarding my first marriage, who do I need to forgive and for what in order to have this be complete?
4. Regarding my first marriage, who do I need to thank in order to be complete?
5. Regarding my first marriage, is there anything else I need to say in order to be complete?

The core of this process is the willingness and ability to forgive. Choosing to forgive makes available enormous energy, which can be used to heal your body and mind and energize you to create the life you want.

The Sedona Method

Negative emotional energy that we suppress in our system can be a significant factor impacting our ability to be well. The Sedona

Method, created by Lester Levenson, is a powerful process that is uniquely designed to release us from negative emotional charge. This energy, once released, can free us into being present to ourselves and to life in a way that supports healing and aliveness. For more information about this powerful technique, please read, *The Sedona Method* by Hale Dwoskin.

Assessing your level of stress

In dealing with stress, the first step is to assess your overall stress level subjectively. Rate your stress level on a scale of 1 to 10. (1 being no stress and 10 being severe stress.) It's important to tell the truth about what you're feeling and experiencing as the starting point.

To get more insight and awareness into how you are experiencing stress, please take the **Self-Assessment Stress Questionnaire** in Addendum D.

Chapter 6

Common Mistakes

The most common mistakes people make when trying to resolve chronic health issues are the following:

1. **Mistake**: We are taught that symptoms are the problem and must be eliminated and yet we are never taught to look for causes of the symptoms.

    Comment: Since the root causes of symptoms are not addressed, these symptoms come back frequently, and repeatedly new symptoms occur as a result of the toxic side effect of medications used in treatment.

2. **Mistake:** Underestimating the compounding negative effect of nutrient deficiencies, toxicity and stress.

    Comment: Consider the impact on your health if you were exposed to several significant levels of toxins such as a statin drug, a mouth full of mercury dental fillings and long term exposure to EMR from a power line. Let's say you were also going through a divorce and you have low levels of zinc and vitamin D in your body. The compounding effect of these factors on your health could be devastating compared to the impact of any one of these factors alone.

3. **Mistake**: Holding the belief that poor health is primarily a result of aging, poor genetics and random exposure to pathogens.

   Comment: This viewpoint encourages us to feel helpless and at the effect of things that one can't control when in fact you can control the vast majority of factors impacting your health.

4. **Mistake**: Giving up too early on implementing the recommendations to address the underlying causes of one's health issues.

   Comment: Many people underestimate the cumulative effect of long-term toxin exposure, nutrient deficiencies and stress. **The general rule of thumb is for every year you have neglected addressing the underlying causes of your health issues, you will need at least one month of conscious application of the principles in this book to remedy your situation.** So if you've been neglecting your health for 20 years, you should expect to see significant improvements in 20 months.

5. **Mistake:** Over-emphasizing infections and under-emphasizing nutrient deficiencies, toxicity and stress in dealing with health issues.

   Comment: Many people have come to see me and have spent months or even years treating candida overgrowth, parasite conditions and viral infections with little success. Once they began to address nutrient deficiencies, toxicities and stress, things improved.

> When Epstein-Barr, Cytomegalovirus, candida and parasite infections ravaged my health in my 20's, I made little or no progress until I got adequate nutrition, substantially reduced my toxic load and reduced my stress levels. I've consistently observed this same phenomenon in my private practice including my four years working at Dr. Mercola's Optimal Wellness Center.

6. **Mistake:** Confusing a "retracing" pattern or detoxification response with an adverse reaction or a set back.

    Comment: Slow down on the program, drink plenty of water and trust that your body knows what to do. All you need to do is give your body what it needs to heal including:

    - Rest and adequate sleep
    - All the nutrients it needs to function properly including water and nutrient-dense whole foods
    - Reducing stress
    - Reducing your toxic load

    It is very important to have patience with yourself and the healing process. Healing is not a linear progression. You may need to go through some ups and downs before you've fully recovered.

7. **Mistake**: Not trusting your body's innate intelligence to heal.

    Comment: The body is programmed to heal and regenerate itself. Look at how your skin heals after a cut, how your hair and nails grow automatically, and how you digest your food without a thought. It is amazing that we overlook this intelligence when we "get sick" or start a decline in health.

8. **Mistake:** Overestimating the nutritional content of your food.

   Comment: Micronutrient deficiencies such as vitamins, minerals and antioxidants are not detectable by most people and we often mistakenly believe that eating organic foods will give us all the nutrients we need.

Chapter 7

Frequently Asked Questions

Q. **What about infections? Aren't they a primary cause of health problems**?

A. After nutrient deficiencies, toxicity and stress; chronic infections (such as candida, parasites, Hepatitis C and Epstein Barr Virus) are often the next most important cause of poor health. The fact is that infections take hold in the body when our immune system is suppressed by nutrient deficiencies (such as vitamins C and D among others), toxicities such as chemicals, heavy metals, radiation and stress.

Q. **What about vaccines? Don't they prevent disease**?

A. I address chronic health conditions more than infectious disease in my practice. My perspective is that building a strong immune system with excellent nutrition, including addressing common nutrient deficiencies and reducing one's toxic load is the best prevention against acute infections. For anyone sincerely interested in researching the effectiveness of vaccines in preventing infectious disease, I recommend reading the books I have listed in the Resource Guide on vaccines. (See Vaccine Safety and Effectiveness in the Resource Guide.)

Q. **What is a detoxification reaction and how do I deal with it?**

A. First, remember that your body has most likely stored a lot of toxins in its fatty tissues, including organs and glands. When you stop eating toxic foods or start a healthier diet, improve your nutritional status or embark on a cleansing program, you will likely start to mobilize some of these stored toxins for elimination. If the channels for eliminating toxins (bowels, kidneys, lungs and skin) are not relatively clear and if your toxic load is significant, you may experience symptoms such as: fatigue, headaches, aches, bowel disturbances or skin outbreaks.

There are 5 Steps to take to mitigate a detoxification reaction:

1. Make sure your bowels are moving at least 2-3 times per day. Use herbal formulas or other colon cleansers if necessary. (See Resource Guide/ Nutritional Supplements.)

2. Increase water intake – filtered, distilled (best to draw out toxins through kidneys) or spring water.

   Remember the adage: "The solution to pollution is dilution"!

3. Take saunas or detox baths to utilize skin as pathway to eliminate toxins.

4. Reduce the dosage of the remedy or formula that is accelerating the detoxification rate. (For many people with chronic health issues, I recommend utilizing the services of a qualified nutrition and detox coach).

5. Remember that your body needs protein to support adequate levels of glutathione, which helps move toxins out of the body and protect cells from damage. Don't fast from all protein even if you need to take a protein

supplement such as a whey protein or a rice protein based formula.

Q. **Can detoxification affect my medications?**

A. Detoxification has the potential to change the way some medicines work. **If you are taking prescription medications then discuss this with your practitioner.** As your level of nutrition improves and your toxic load decreases, many people are able to either reduce the dose of their prescription medication or stop taking the medication entirely. **I must emphasize that you should always consult your doctor about whether or not to reduce your medication dose.**

Q. **What are your top recommendations to prevent illness and keep healthy?** I don't have any major health problems but want to stay healthy, feel more energetic and reduce the chance of developing a serious health condition.

A. Here are my top seven recommendations:

1. **Make sure you get proper nutrition** by following a good diet focusing on: high quality protein, organic vegetables and healthy fats. Reduce grains; avoid processed foods, sugar, sweets and caffeine, moderation with alcohol preferably organic, red wine. Take a **whole-food multivitamin**/mineral supplement or a high quality liquid vitamin/mineral supplement like Dr. Drucker's *All in One* liquid supplement to cover potential deficiencies. (See Resource Guide/Nutritional Supplements).

2. **Make sure your bowels are moving on average 2 to 3 times per day.** This is accomplished by

addressing: adequate hydration; good lev*els of healthy bacteria in* your intestines with high quality yogurt, other cultured foods or a good pro-biotic supplement; a diet high in fiber (plenty of fresh fruits and vegetables, whole grains, raw nuts and seeds); making sure you have adequate levels of magnesium which is essential for healthy bowel functions. A toxic bowel is the starting point of many health problems. If necessary take herbal formula or other colon cleansing products to get your bowels moving. I have found OxyPowder to be especially helpful. (See Resource Guide products section.)

3. **Physical movement is critical for health.** Ideally you would take long brisk walks in nature and get plenty of fresh air and sunshine and connect to the earth. Consistent moderate exercise is great and preferably outdoors as often as possible.

4. **Prioritize connecting to spirit** in whatever way you are inclined. If you have no reference point for this, spend time in nature alone and with no specific intention other than to let yourself feel part of the natural world.

5. **Get adequate rest.** Build into your life daily, weekly, monthly and yearly breaks away from work and stressful situations. Weekend trips and periodic vacations always work well when we experience a dip in our health or vitality. Even when I could not afford a week vacation I would turn off the phone, shut down the computer and sit quietly in my backyard or create a vacation experience in my own home. Remember, adequate sleep is critical to restore your energy and to support toxin removal from your brain.

6. **Increase activities, which boost oxytocin levels.** The "cuddle hormone" is one of the best antidotes to

high levels of stress hormones such as cortisol. Positive social interactions with friends and family, healing and nurturing touch and conscious sexual intimacy are great stress reducing activities.

7. **Avoid toxic substances such as** toxic cleaners, GMO foods and foods sprayed with pesticides. Be sure to remove mercury dental fillings and filter your drinking and bathing water from toxic chemicals and heavy metals. I recommend reading, *Our Toxic World: A Wake Up Call,* by Dr. Doris Rapp.

Q. If I do have a chronic infection (bacterial, viral, candida, fungal or parasite), what is the best way to address it?

A. Here are my top six recommendations to deal with chronic infections:

1. Strengthen your immune system with good nutrition and stress reduction. Vitamins C and D boost your immune system. Get more rest and laugh – both important for the immune system.

2. Use a high quality pro-biotic to improve digestion and elimination and support liver detoxification. This will clear the gut and blood of toxins and pathogens. A toxic blood stream and toxic cells are a breeding ground for infections. **Think of what grows in a garbage can if you don't empty it – maggots!**

3. Take natural antimicrobial herbs and plants: raw garlic, onions, oregano, herbs like cats claw, pau d'arco and jatoba are legendary for clearing out chronic infections. These herbs are highly beneficial for the immune and endocrine systems as well.

4. Do a series of saunas. Infrared or far infrared saunas trigger your body to clear out toxins and pathogens by sweating them out through the skin, our largest detoxification pathway.

5. Take systemic enzymes on an empty stomach. These enzymes break down toxins, bacteria and support immune function. (See Resource Guide supplement section.)

6. "Oil pulling" is an ancient ayurvedic therapy to clear up allergies, sinus and upper respiratory infections and systemic candida infections. I personally do it almost daily to improve oral and gastrointestinal health as well as to support general detoxification.

   Follow these instructions to perform the oil pulling method:

   - Oil pulling should be done on an empty stomach (preferably first thing in the morning).
   - Use one tablespoon of either organic extra virgin coconut oil or organic sesame oil.
   - Swish the oil around your mouth slowly and be sure that the oil reaches all parts of your mouth – DO NOT swallow.
   - Swish for between 5-20 minutes. Start with five minutes and work your way up to twenty minutes.
   - Spit out all of the oil when you are done and rinse your mouth with water and brush your teeth with natural, fluoride free toothpaste afterwards.

     Note: Some people may feel tired, nauseous or have other flu-like symptoms after oil pulling. This is generally a good sign that your body is removing toxins and pathogens and will subside when you are healthier.

Conclusion

We all want and deserve to be healthy, but most of us don't understand how our every day choices impact the level of well being that we experience. Much of our suffering both physical and emotional can be avoided if we understand how the **Underlying Causation Paradigm** operates in our lives. By embracing this new paradigm, as I have described in this book, we can naturally apply sound principles of nutrition, regular detoxification strategies and stress reduction that insure good health. With a deeper understanding of what causes illness, we can build a solid foundation for a lifetime of vibrant health.

When my physical and emotional health deteriorated in my early 20's, I found myself at a crossroads. Would I succumb to cynicism, despair and failed conventional approaches for treating symptoms, or would I look deep within for the strength to do what was necessary to truly heal? It took time for me to understand everything I needed to know before my health would improve, but with patience and persistence, I not only retrieved my health, but I also gained a profound understanding of the causes of my illness.

In closing, I want to tell you a short story about a client I had in Chicago. My client, whom I will call Jane, came to me with a laundry list of symptoms including the following: chronic fatigue, hypothyroidism, insomnia, constipation and depression. When she came to my office, she told me that nothing was working with her body. She gave me a list of her symptoms and complaints, and after listening for a few minutes I looked her in the eye and said,

"I know you think that nothing in your body works right, but I don't believe you. I saw you walk in to my office and noticed that your legs work just fine. I noticed that you weren't wearing glasses. Do you wear glasses?"

Conclusion

"No," she said, "I have perfect eyesight".

I proceeded to question her about all of the aspects of her health that appeared to be working well for her. At this point, she started to cry and said,

"You're right, I am basically a healthy person and I still need your help."

"Great," I said. "Your willingness to acknowledge what's already working is our starting point."

Don't get me wrong, this woman was clearly suffering from toxic overload, but her health would improve faster if she focused on becoming ever more healthy and not exclusively on getting rid of her illnesses. Please remember that regardless of your current condition, you always have some level of health to acknowledge and appreciate, and that is the best place to begin.

Jane then asked for a list of the top 50 things to do for her health over the next year. I wrote up a list of 50 things to do to improve her health including: getting her mercury dental fillings safely replaced with non-toxic substances; doing a colon cleanse every three months; doing a liver cleanse and a heavy metal cleanse; eating only organic food; getting filters for her tap water and shower head. I also recommended that she do some work around forgiveness and get in touch with what brought her joy in addition to being more patient and compassionate with herself.

After this appointment, I didn't see Jane for a long time. It was nearly a year later when she finally came to see me again. When she did return, I noticed immediately how well she looked. She told me that she had done all 50 things I had recommended to her and that she felt even better than she did before she got sick. She realized that she had to stop feeling resigned about her lack of health and start taking responsibility for retrieving her well-being with an open mind. She made a commitment to herself and put into action the principles of the **Underlying Causation Paradigm** taught in this book.

We each have points in our lives when we are given an opportunity to make a course correction in our favor. Many of my clients over the years have come to me after exhausting conventional medical approaches to their health issues and other less comprehensive natural healing approaches. The conventional medical paradigm, which emphasizes treating symptoms with medication, gives you very little control over the long-term quality of your health.

There is no substitute for knowledge when it comes to maintaining and improving your health. This includes understanding how your body works and what it needs to function optimally. It also includes understanding what depletes your body and impairs its ability to function properly. This book is an invitation to implement the **Underlying Causation Paradigm** in your life and give yourself the gift of vibrant health.

Addendum A: Resource Guide

Education

Electromagnetic Field Impact on Health

www.electromagnetichealth.org – Research and Education on the impact of EMFs on health.

Food and Nutrition

www.helpguide.org/life/organic_foods_pesticides_gmo.htm – education regarding organic vs. non-organic food, health benefits of organic food and more.

www.organicconsumers.org/articles/article_28779.cfm – research on nutrient content of organic vs. non-organic food.

www.small-farm-permaculture-and-sustainable-living.com – How to grown your own organic food and live sustainably.

www.westonaprice.org – Nutrition, food and farming education

Health and Wellness Education

www.createvibranthealth.com

www.drlwilson.com

www.enzymeessentials.com

www.mercola.com

www.metabolichhealing.com

www.naturalnews.com

Mercury free dentistry

www.amalgamillness.com

www.iaomt.org

www.savypatients.com/amalgam

Nutrition and Wellness Consultation

www.createvibranthealth.com

www.healthexcel.com (Metabolic Typing)

Professional Training

www.biomedx.com – Live Blood Cell Analysis Training

www.healthexcel.com (Metabolic Typing)

www.metabolichhealing.com

www.drlwilson.com Hair mineral analysis research and information.

Vaccine Research

www.nvic.org – National Vaccine Information Center.

Recommended Reading

Nutrition

- *Nourishing Traditions* by Sally Fallon. Great Nutrition and recipe book with focus on health benefits of animal products and saturated fats.
- *The Body Ecology Diet: Recovering Your Health and Rebuilding Your Immunity* by Donna Gates.
- *Metabolic Typing* by William Wolcott.

- *Grain Brain* by David Perlmutter, MD. The adverse effects of high carbohydrate foods and diets on brain health.
- *The Handbook of Intermittent Fasting – Effective Solutions for Weight Loss & Muscle Definition* by Idai Makay
- *Your Body's Many Cries for Water: You Are Not Sick, You Are Thirsty!* By Fereydoon Batmanghelidj
- *Iodine: Why you need it, Why you can't live without it* by Dr. David Brownstein
- *Alternative Medicine: The Definitive Guide* by Burton Goldberg.

Stress and Emotional Healing

- *The Power of Now* by Eckhart Tolle
- *The Sedona Method* by Hale Dwoskin
- *Earthing* by Ober, Sinatra and Zucker.

Toxicity

- *Excitotoxins: The Taste that Kills* by Russell Blaylock, MD
- *The Hundred Year Lie: How chemicals destroy the immune system* by Randall Fitzgerald
- *Our Toxic World: A Wake Up Call* by Dr. Doris Rapp
- *Cell Phones: Invisible Hazards in the Wireless Age: An Insider's Alarming Discoveries* by Dr. George Carlo
- *The Green Beauty Guide: Your Essential Resource to Organic and Natural Skin Care, Hair Care, Makeup, and Fragrances* by Julie Gabriel.

Vaccine Safety and Effectiveness

- *Vaccine Safety Manual for Concerned Families and Health Practitioners, 2nd Edition: Guide to Immunization Risks and Protection* by Neil Miller.

- *Dissolving Illusions: Disease, Vaccines and the Forgotten History* by Suzanne Humphries, MD.

Nutritional Supplements and other Health Care Products

Colon cleanses, Probiotics and digestive health

- Oxy-Powder colon cleanse. www.globalhealigcenter.com
- Intestinal formula #1. www.herbdoc.com
- LB17 – Live culture probiotic. www.osumex.com
- CytoFlora® – cell wall lysed probiotic. www.bioray.com
- Digest Gold – high quality full spectrum digestive enzyme. www.enzymedica.com

Detoxification programs

- D-Toxol, D-Toxol Accelerator and Children's D-Toxol by Ultra Life. www.ultralifeinc.com
- Liver Life®, NDF® and NDF Plus®. Liver cleanse and heavy metal/chemical detoxification formula. www.bioray.com
- Chem Detox. Pectin product. www.prllabs.com
- Perfect Cleanse. www.gardenoflife.com
- Cleanse Smart. www.renwlife.com

- Serracore NK, Exclzyme systemic enzymes. www.astenzymes.com
- Custom detoxification clay and essential oil baths for different toxicities. www.magneticclay.com
- High quality clay detoxification products as well as herbal cleansing formulas. www.vitalityherbsandclay.com

EMR remediation

- Tools and technologies to reduce adverse health effects of EMR. www.lessemf.com
- Testing, tools and technologies to reduce adverse health effects of EMR. www.emfsse.com
- Earthing is a fast-growing movement based upon the major discovery that connecting to the Earth's natural energy is foundational for vibrant health. www.earthing.com

Green Super Food Formulas

- Nano Greens and other powerful whole food supplements. www.biopharmasci.com

Medicinal Herbal formulas

- Amazon rainforest herbal extracts and formulas for infections and rejuvenation. www.raintreeformulas.com

Organ and glandular regeneration

- Drenamin, Thytrophin, renafood, livaplex and other protomorphogen gland extracts. www.standprocess.com
- Laminine a whole food protein adaptogen which activates dormant stem cells to regenerate weakened organs and glands. www.supportforyourbody.com

Other health related products

- Comparison for top water filters and air purifiers. www.allergybuyersclub.com
- Scalar wave lasers and other products. www.supportforyourbody.com

Testing

- Hair Tissue Mineral Analysis (HTMA) – the best website on the value of HTMA. www.drlwilson.com
- Blood testing including vitamins, minerals, amino acids, kidney and liver function, hormone levels and more. www.lef.org/bloodtest
- Blood tests. www.doctorsdata.com
- Recommended labs for HTMA Analytical research labs – www.arltma.com; and Trace Elements www.traceelements.com

Whole Food Vitamin/Mineral supplements

- Garden of Life, www.gardenoflife.com
- New Chapter, www.newchapter.com
- Innate Response, www.innateresponse.com
- Dr. Druckers Labs, www.store.druckerlabs.com

Addendum B: Vitamins, their functions in the body and their sources

Vitamins are used to produce energy and synthesize tissues, enzymes, hormones and other vital compounds. The table below groups vitamins into those soluble in fat and those soluble in water and provides major functions and sources of vitamins.

VITAMIN	FUNCTION	SOURCES
Fat-Soluble Vitamins		
Vitamin A	Promotes normal growth of bones, growth and repair of body tissues; bone and tooth formation; vision; antioxidant in the form of beta-carotene	Milk, butter, dairy products, dark green vegetables, yellow-orange fruits and vegetables
Vitamin D	Regulates absorption and use of calcium and phosphorus; aids in building and maintaining bones and teeth	Direct exposure of the skin to sunlight, fortified milk, margarine, eggs, liver, fish

Vitamin E	Protects red blood cells; antioxidant (protects fat-soluble vitamins); stabilizes cell membranes	Vegetable oils, dark green leafy vegetables, nuts, legumes, egg yolks, salad dressings, mayonnaise, wheat germ, whole grains
Vitamin K	Required for synthesis of blood-clotting proteins	Bacterial synthesis in digestive tract, dark green leafy vegetables, liver, milk, grain products, egg yolk

Water-Soluble Vitamins

Vitamin C (ascorbic acid)	Plays an important role in collagen formation (helps heal wounds, maintains bones and teeth, strengthens blood vessels); antioxidant; strengthens resistance to infection and helps body absorb iron	Citrus fruits and juices, tomatoes, potatoes, dark green vegetables, peppers, lettuce, cantaloupe, strawberries, mangoes, papayas, cauliflower
Vitamin B1 (thiamin)	Helps enzymes release energy from carbohydrates	Meat, pork, liver, fish, poultry, whole-grain and enriched breads, cereals, legumes, nuts, green leafy vegetables
Vitamin B2 (riboflavin)	Helps enzymes release energy from carbohydrates, protein and fat; promotes healthy skin and good vision	Milk, cheese, yogurt, enriched breads and cereals, green leafy vegetables, fish, liver, lean meats, yeast

Addendum B: Vitamins, their functions in the body and their sources

Niacin (nicotinic acid)	Helps enzymes release energy from carbohydrates, protein and fat; promotes healthy skin, nerves and digestive system	Yeast, whole grains and enriched breads and cereals, milk, meats, nuts, legumes, peanuts
Folate (folic acid)	Required for red blood cell formation, new cell division, protein metabolism	Dark green leafy vegetables, citrus fruits, enriched grains and cereals, legumes, seeds, melons, yeast, orange juice, asparagus
Vitamin B6 (pyridoxine)	Required for amino acid metabolism; used in protein and fat metabolism; aids in forming red blood cells and antibodies	Dark green leafy vegetables, whole-grain products, meats, liver, poultry, fish, shellfish, soybeans, wheat germ, fruits
Vitamin B12 (cobalamin)	Necessary for normal growth; helps maintain nerve cells and red blood cells; aids in synthesis of genetic materials	Primarily in animal products meat, fish, poultry, liver, eggs, milk and milk products, fortified cereals
Biotin	Coenzyme in energy metabolism; glycogen formation; fat synthesis	Legumes, egg yolks, chocolate, cauliflower, yeast, liver, nuts, milk

Pantothenic acid	Component of coenzyme for energy metabolism	Legumes, whole grains, lean beef, milk, potatoes, yeast, egg yolks, liver, peanuts, tomatoes, broccoli, fish, poultry; small amounts in fruits and vegetable

Addendum C

Minerals: functions in the body and sources

A mineral is defined as inorganic element containing no carbon that remains as ash when food is burned. Although as many as 40 minerals are in existence, the table below describes the 17 minerals that are essential to human nutrition and lists their functions and sources in food.

MINERAL	FUNCTION	SOURCES
Macrominerals		
Calcium	Strengthens bones and teeth; involved in muscle contraction and relaxation, blood clotting, water balance, nerve function	Milk and milk products, green leafy vegetables, legumes, fortified foods, almonds, fish (with bones), tofu
Phosphorus	Involved in calcification of teeth and bones, acid-base balance, energy metabolism	Meat, poultry, fish, milk, soft drinks, processed foods, whole grains, eggs
Sodium	Promotes acid-base balance, water balance, nerve impulse transmission, muscle activity	Salt, soy sauce, processed foods: cured, canned, pickled and many prepackaged foods

Potassium	Facilitates many reactions, especially protein synthesis, water balance, nerve transmission, muscle contraction	Meats, milk, fruits, vegetables, grains, legumes
Sulfur	Component of protein; part of biotin, thiamin, insulin	All protein-containing foods
Chloride	Part of stomach acid, acid base balance, water balance	Table salt, soy sauce; processed foods
Magnesium	Involved in protein synthesis, muscle contraction, nerve transmission	Whole grains, nuts, legumes, chocolate, meat, dark green leafy vegetables, seafoods, cocoa
Microminerals		
Iron	Hemoglobin formation, part of myoglobin in muscles; used in energy utilization	Red meats, fish, poultry, shellfish, eggs, legumes, dried fruits, fortified cereals and grains
Iodine	Part of thyroxine, a thyroid hormone that influences growth and metabolism	Iodized salt, seafood, seaweed, bread
Zinc	Part of insulin and enzymes; vitamin A transport; wound healing; fetus and sperm development; immunity;	Protein-containing foods: red meat, seafood, oysters, clams, poultry, eggs, dairy, grains

Addendum C: Minerals, their functions in the body and their sources

	promotes enzyme activity and metabolism	
Selenium	Antioxidant; works with vitamin E; immune system response	Seafood, meats, grains
Manganese	Essential for normal bone development; activates enzymes	Whole grains, legumes, nuts, green leafy vegetables, meat, tea, coffee
Copper	Necessary for formation of hemoglobin; part of energy metabolism enzymes	Organ meats, shellfish, nuts, seeds, legumes, peanut butter, chocolate
Fluoride	Formation of bones and teeth; provides resistance to dental caries	Naturally occurring in drinking water vs. drinking water where sodium fluoride (a toxic by-product) has been added, tea, seafood
Chromium	Enhances effect of insulin; aids in metabolism of carbohydrates and lipids	Mushrooms, dark chocolate, prunes, nuts, asparagus, brewer's yeast, whole grains, vegetable oils
Molybdenum	Aids in oxidation reactions	Legumes, cereals, grains, organ meats
Cobalt	As part of vitamin B12, aids in nerve function and blood formation	Meats, milk and milk products

Addendum D

Detoxification Program

This program can be done anywhere from 7 to 28 days. It is always better to start slow to see how your body responds to a detoxification program. For those on medication or who have serious health problems you should consult a health care professional who has experience in coaching people in detoxification.

Basic 7-Day Detox Program:

Cut out all sweets, caffeine, alcohol, processed foods and sugar.

Cut out dairy products, red meat and all refined grains.

Eat fruits, vegetables, nuts, seeds, beans, legumes, whole grains such as brown rice, beans, quinoa, amaranth, eggs and free-range poultry or wild caught fish.

Note: If weight loss is desired, cut out grains and starchy vegetables like potatoes, yams, beets and carrots.

Essential Components of Detoxification Program:

1. Drink approximately half your body weight (measured in pounds) in ounces of pure water per day. Add fresh squeezed lemon to several of the glasses of water.

2. Only eat organic foods if possible. Add foods and herbs to improve circulation, digestion and elimination such as garlic, red clover, ginger and cayenne pepper to meals.

3. Moderate exercise – walking, rebounding, light workouts.

4. Drink either 12 ounces of fresh vegetable juice per day (more greens in general is better) or make your own if you have a juicer or buy one at a juice bar; or if you don't have a juicer and can't get to a juice bar use a green super-food formula. I use 1 Tablespoon in a 12 oz. glass per day. Excellent choices include: Perfect food from Garden of Life, Green Vibrance by Vibrant Health or NanoGreens by BioPharma Scientific (my personal favorite).

Here are some optional enhancements to the Detoxification Program if you go beyond 7 days:

A. Take a high quality whole body cleansing program supplement such as: Renew Life's Cleanse Smart; or Garden of Life's Perfect Cleanse; or the Heavy Metal/Chemical detoxification program (listed in B. below) but DO NOT do both at the same time. One option is to do a full body cleanse first, wait 2-4 weeks and then proceed to the Heavy Metal/Chemical Detoxification program.

B. Heavy metal/chemical detoxification program. There are two programs I recommend for my clients. These programs are a bit more expensive and do a better job at cleansing toxins which have accumulated at the cellular level.*

- BIORAY® has a three part program which includes a Liver/Kidney cleansing formula called Liver Life®, a very high quality probiotic, CytoFlora® and a chemical/heavy metal/radiation detox formula, NDF® and NDF

Plus®. For more information on this program go to www.bioray.com (Use the coupon code JORDAN to receive 10% off all purchases.)

- I also recommend a formula by Ultra Life called D-Toxol. For more information on this product go to www.ultralifeinc.com

*If you do better with liquids go with the BIORAY® program since all formulas are liquid and can be dosed at very low starting points if you are sensitive. If convenience and ability to travel while on your detox program are your priorities, I recommend using D-Toxol since it is in capsule form and is easier for traveling.

If at any point during a cleanse you experience headaches, extreme fatigue, bloating, gas, muscle pain or any other aggravation of your symptoms incorporate some or all of following steps:

- Make sure your bowels are moving at least 2-3 x day. Use herbal formulas or other colon cleansers such as OxyPowder if necessary. (See Resource Guide supplement section.)

- Increase water intake – filtered, distilled (best to draw out toxins through kidneys) or spring water. **Remember the adage – "the solution to pollution is dilution!"**

- Take saunas or detox baths to utilize skin as pathway to eliminate toxins.

- Reduce the dosage of the remedy or formula that is accelerating the detoxification rate.

- Remember that your body needs protein to support adequate levels of Glutathione, which helps move toxins out of the body and protect cells from damage.

Take a protein supplement such as a whey protein or a rice protein based formula.

Optimizing your body's capacity to eliminate heavy metals and chemicals will put you on the fast track to vibrant health. I recommend incorporating detoxification programs (for a minimum of 7 days) into your overall health program at least once every six months and optimally once a season.

Forms and Surveys

DAILY DIET DIARY: Learning to Listen to Your Body

BREAKFAST
How was your mood before breakfast?
What did you have for Breakfast?
Time:
BEFORE LUNCH ASSESSMENT OF BREAKFAST
Was your breakfast satisfying to you?
Did you need a snack before lunch?
Did you or do you have any cravings?
How is your energy?
How is your mood?
How is your mental clarity?
What did you have for Lunch?
Time:
BEFORE DINNER ASSESSMENT OF LUNCH
Was lunch satisfying to you?
Did you need a snack before dinner?
Did you or do you have any cravings?
How is your energy?
How is your mood?
How is your mental clarity?
What did you have for Dinner?
Time:
BEFORE BEDTIME ASSESSMENT OF DINNER
Was dinner satisfying to you?
Did you need a snack before dinner?
Did you or do you have any cravings?
How is your mood?
Did you need a snack between dinner and bedtime?
Did you or do you have any cravings?
How is your mood?

What is your overall assessment of how you felt today on a scale of 1 to 10?
(1 being extremely poor; 10 being excellent)

Forms and Surveys

TOXICITY QUESTIONNAIRE

Rate each of the following based upon your health profile of the last 90 days.

0	Rarely or never experience the symptom
1	Occasionally experience the symptom – effect is not severe
2	Occasionally experience the symptom – effect is severe
3	Frequently experience the symptom – effect is not severe
4	Frequently experience the symptom – effect is severe

1. DIGESTIVE   Total: ____

a.	Nausea and/or vomiting	0	1	2	3	4
b.	Diarrhea	0	1	2	3	4
c.	Constipation	0	1	2	3	4
d.	Bloated Feeling	0	1	2	3	4
e.	Belching and/or passing gas	0	1	2	3	4
f.	Heartburn	0	1	2	3	4

2. EARS   Total: ____

a.	Itchy ears	0	1	2	3	4
b.	Earaches and ear infections	0	1	2	3	4
c.	Drainage from ear	0	1	2	3	4
d.	Ringing in ears	0	1	2	3	4
e.	Hearing Loss	0	1	2	3	4

3. EMOTIONS   Total: ____

a.	Mood swings	0	1	2	3	4
b.	Anxiety/fear/nervousness	0	1	2	3	4
c.	Anger/irritability	0	1	2	3	4
d.	Depression	0	1	2	3	4
e.	Sense of despair	0	1	2	3	4
f.	Uncaring or disinterested	0	1	2	3	4

4. ENERGY/ACTIVITY   Total: ____

a.	Fatigue or sluggishness	0	1	2	3	4
b.	Hyperactivity	0	1	2	3	4
c.	Restlessness	0	1	2	3	4
d.	Insomnia	0	1	2	3	4
e.	Startled awake at night	0	1	2	3	4

5. EYES   Total: ____

a.	Watery or itchy eyes	0	1	2	3	4
b.	Swollen, red or sticky eyelids	0	1	2	3	4
c.	Dark circles under eyes	0	1	2	3	4
d.	Blurred or tunnel vision	0	1	2	3	4

6. HEAD   Total:

a.	Headaches	0	1	2	3	4
b.	Faintness	0	1	2	3	4
c.	Dizziness	0	1	2	3	4
d.	Pressure	0	1	2	3	4

7. LUNGS   Total:

a.	Chest congestion	0	1	2	3	4
b.	Asthma or bronchitis	0	1	2	3	4
c.	Shortness or breath	0	1	2	3	4
d.	Difficulty breathing	0	1	2	3	4

8. MIND   Total:

a.	Poor Memory	0	1	2	3	4
b.	Confusion	0	1	2	3	4
c.	Poor concentration	0	1	2	3	4
d.	Poor coordination	0	1	2	3	4
e.	Difficulty breathing	0	1	2	3	4
f.	Difficulty making decisions	0	1	2	3	4
g.	Stuttering/stammering	0	1	2	3	4
h.	Slurred speech	0	1	2	3	4
i.	Learning disabilities	0	1	2	3	4

9. MOUTH/THROAT   Total:

a.	Chronic coughing	0	1	2	3	4
b.	Gagging	0	1	2	3	4
c.	Frequent need to clear throat	0	1	2	3	4
d.	Swollen or discolored tongue, gums, lips	0	1	2	3	4
e.	Canker sores	0	1	2	3	4

10. NOSE   Total:

a.	Stuffy nose	0	1	2	3	4
b.	Sinus problems	0	1	2	3	4
c.	Hay fever	0	1	2	3	4
d.	Sneezing attacks	0	1	2	3	4
e.	Excessive mucous	0	1	2	3	4

11. SKIN Total: _____

a.	Acne	0	1	2	3	4
b.	Hives, rashes, dry skin	0	1	2	3	4
c.	Hair loss	0	1	2	3	4
d.	Flushing	0	1	2	3	4
e.	Excessive sweating	0	1	2	3	4

12. HEART Total: _____

a.	Skipped heartbeats	0	1	2	3	4
b.	Rapid heartbeats	0	1	2	3	4
c.	Chest pain	0	1	2	3	4

13. JOINTS/MUSCLES Total: _____

a.	Pain or aches in joints	0	1	2	3	4
b.	Rheumatoid arthritis	0	1	2	3	4
c.	Osteoarthritis	0	1	2	3	4
d.	Stiffness/limited movement	0	1	2	3	4
e.	Pain or aches in muscles	0	1	2	3	4
f.	Recurrent back aches	0	1	2	3	4
g.	Feeling weakness or tiredness	0	1	2	3	4

14. WEIGHT Total: _____

a.	Binge eating or drinking	0	1	2	3	4
b.	Craving certain foods	0	1	2	3	4
c.	Excessive weight	0	1	2	3	4
d.	Compulsive eating	0	1	2	3	4
e.	Water retention	0	1	2	3	4
f.	Underweight	0	1	2	3	4

15. OTHER Total: _____

a.	Frequent illness	0	1	2	3	4
b.	Frequent or urgent urination	0	1	2	3	4
c.	Leaky bladder	0	1	2	3	4
d.	Genital itch or discharge	0	1	2	3	4

Grand Total: _____

If your score is 0 – 20, your body is functioning very well and you probably don't need to do a detox program immediately.

If your score is 21 – 40, toxins are building up and you would be advised to do at least a short 7-day detoxification program.

If your score is 41 – 60, you are toxic and whatever health issues you have will only get worse if you do not make a concerted effort to reduce your toxic load now.

If your score is over 60, you will probably need professional coaching to improve your health and a period of building up your health may be necessary before starting a more comprehensive detoxification program.

Note: See Addendum **for Detox Program Guidelines.**

Self-Assessment Stress Questionnaire

		Often	Sometimes	Rarely
1	Do you find that you are easily irritated?			
2	Do you bring work home at night?			
3	Do you feel that there are not enough hour in the day to do all the things you must do?			
4	Do you suffer from tension headaches?			
5	Do you feel tired and have no energy even after a good night's sleep?			
6	Are you physically tense?			
7	Do your muscles ache?			
8	Do you grind your teeth at night?			
9	Do you suffer from insomnia?			
10	Do you feel overwhelmed?			
11	Do you lack self confidence?			
12	Do you feel dissatisfied with your life?			
13	Do you experienced mood swings?			
14	Do you experience difficultly making decisions?			
15	Do you pretend to be listening to others even though you are preoccupied with your own thoughts?			
16	Do you drink alcohol to relax?			
17	Do you find yourself using caffeine to start the day?			
18	Are your relationships with people strained and difficult?			
19	Do you feel dissatisfied with your work?			
20	Do you feel dissatisfied with your home life?			
21	Do you worry?			
22	Is it difficult for you to relax?			
23	Do you find that you don't have time for your hobbies and interests?			
24	Are you impatient?			
25	Do you drive, talk or walk quickly?			

Scoring

If you answered "**Always**", give yourself 2 points.

If you answered "**Sometimes**", give yourself 1 point.

If you answered "**Rarely or Never**", give yourself 0 point.

0-15: You are not particularly stressed and are coping well with the stress you have or you are not aware of much stress in your life.

15-25: You are probably moderately stressed and would benefit from implementing some of the top seven stress reduction tips in Chapter 6.

25-50: You are probably experiencing a significant level of stress. I would prioritize the stress reduction tips in Chapter 6 and make sure to include nutritional support for your adrenal glands including: adaptogen herbs, B complex vitamins. I would also strongly recommend taking a break from stressful situations for a while until you can get your score down. Also, a vacation may be in order.

Made in the USA
Middletown, DE
21 October 2017

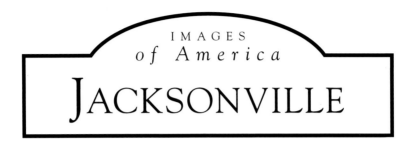

Margaret LaPlante and the
Southern Oregon Historical Society

Copyright © 2010 by Margaret LaPlante and the Southern Oregon Historical Society
ISBN 978-0-7385-8055-5

Published by Arcadia Publishing
Charleston SC, Chicago IL, Portsmouth NH, San Francisco CA

Printed in the United States of America

Library of Congress Control Number: 2010920201

For all general information contact Arcadia Publishing at:
Telephone 843-853-2070
Fax 843-853-0044
E-mail sales@arcadiapublishing.com
For customer service and orders:
Toll-Free 1-888-313-2665

Visit us on the Internet at www.arcadiapublishing.com

This book is dedicated to Alice Hanley and the Hanley sisters, Claire, Martha, and Mary, all of whom played a significant role in preserving the valley's history.

CONTENTS

Acknowledgments 6

Introduction 7

1. The Early Years 9
2. The Chinese and Other Minorities 57
3. The Later Years 73

ACKNOWLEDGMENTS

Today's technology makes it possible for nearly everyone to take photographs. When the photographs in this book were taken, photography was in its infancy. Very few people were trained in the field of photography and fewer had the required equipment. Those who were skilled in photography generally moved from town to town in order to make a living. There simply wasn't enough call for their services in one area, so they were constantly on the move. The history of Jacksonville is all the richer for the talents of one man, Peter Britt. As a young man, Peter immigrated to America from Switzerland with his father and brother. Peter was already a skilled portrait and landscape painter. He soon learned of the new field of Daguerreotype photography and went to St. Louis in 1847 to apprentice under J. H. Fitzsimmons, a leader in the field of photography. When Peter heard of the new country out west, he decided to cross the plains to Oregon. He and two other men rode horseback pulling a wagon. Inside the wagon, Peter had carefully wrapped 300 pounds of his fragile and expensive photography equipment. He settled in Jacksonville in 1852 and soon after, began capturing images of his new community. Those images were preserved by Peter and his children. When his daughter, Mollie, passed away, she left the collection to the Oregon State Higher Board of Education. They have generously shared the collection with the Southern Oregon Historical Society. Within the collection of the Southern Oregon Historical Society are thousands of images of early day Jacksonville. Some of those historic images are shared in this book to provide a glimpse of life in early Jacksonville. All images in this volume appear courtesy of the Southern Oregon Historical Society.

Introduction

The primary tribe of Native Americans in the Rogue Valley was the Takelma Indians. They occupied the land and went about their lives undisturbed except for the occasional fur trapper or explorer who passed through. One group of fur trappers had some trouble with the Takelma Indians and referred to them as "Rogues" and soon the valley took on that name. They were divided into the Upland and Lowland Takelmas.

The Takelma women wore knee-length deerskin shirts adorned with fringe of white grass. The men wore deerskin shirts and leggings tied with a belt, deerskin robes, and blankets and hats made from deerskin or bearskin. They lined their moccasins with grass or fur. During the cold months, they wore sleeves made from fox skins all the way to their hands. They embellished their garments with abalone and other shells, white grass braids, and buckskin tassels.

They wove baskets from tree roots, vines, and other natural resources. The baskets were used for food gathering, food preparation, and serving. They also wove baskets to carry their infants. They had the skill to weave baskets so tightly that they could carry water in them.

Trading with other tribes allowed them to obtain unique items that were not available to them otherwise. The diet of the Takelma Indians consisted of sugar pine nuts and the bark from the sugar pine tree, wild berries and plums, seeds from other trees and plants, and edible plants that grew naturally. They would shell acorns and then mash them using a mortar and pestle. They would then place the mashed acorns on clean sand and pour hot water over them to leach them. That process was repeated, and the mixture was boiled by placing it into a tightly woven basket filled with water and heating it over hot stones. Camas bulbs were baked in a pit dug in the ground. They would place alder bark between the hot stones in the pit and the bulbs. They would cook the bulbs for a day or two until they were roasted. They could then mash them into cakes and store them for the cold months. The river and creeks were full of salmon and trout. The men found plenty of hunting opportunities for deer and elk.

The Takelmas lived in what were referred to as "Pitt houses." They dug down 18 to 24 inches, the length and width of the house, then erected posts in the corners. They used planks from sugar pine trees for the exterior siding and the roof. Other times the roofing was made entirely from what was available from their natural resources. Most villages also had a sweathouse for the men. They heated the sweathouses by pouring water over large stones that had been heated in a fire then brought into the structure. The men utilized the sweathouses for training and purification.

Legend has it that in the spring, the snow on Mt. Pitt (now known as Mt. McLaughlin) would begin to melt. As the snow melted, the wings of an angel would appear in the snow that remained on the mountain. When that happened, it was the perfect time to fish for salmon. Fishing was done by hook and line using a bone connected with sinew. Crawfish was used as bait. They also used long nets to catch fish. Salmon could be traded for animal skins. The natural resources of the Takelma Indians were threatened in the early 1850s as more and more white settlers arrived in the valley. The land they knew was disappearing. Tensions began running high between the two groups. Attacks became commonplace with many deaths resulting. Each party claimed that the attack was completely unprovoked. The whites claimed the Takelmas were attacking them as they made their way into the valley and the Takelmas claimed the whites were attacking them and shooting the tribe with their guns.

The early pioneers of the 1840s found most Native Americans along the Oregon Trail to be friendly and accommodating. There was a language barrier, but they made do with a few simple signals and words. Some Native Americans made a living helping the pioneers cross the treacherous rivers. Others traded with the whites for items that benefitted them both. As the years passed and the number of pioneers increased, the Takelmas resented the erosion of the land they had called home for many years. Their hunting, fishing, and natural vegetation suffered and they began to strike back. When the fighting became too much, many whites went to live with neighbors who had built forts surrounding their homes. They stayed there until it was safe to return home.

In 1853, after many deaths on both sides, Gen. Joseph Lane was sent from up north by the territorial governor of Oregon to help both sides reach a peaceful agreement. Capt. James W. Nesmith accompanied General Lane and a dozen other men on the journey. He later wrote about the experience saying, "After a toilsome march, dragging the howitzer and other materials of war through the Umpqua Canyon and up and down the mountain trails made slippery by recent rains, we arrived at General Lane's encampment on [the] Rogue River."

General Lane made arrangements to meet with the Takelma Indians at their encampment on September 10, 1853. The agreement was that General Lane could bring 10 of his own men, all unarmed, to meet with the Takelmas and their chiefs, Old Jo, John, and Sam. The general and his men were greatly outnumbered, but undeterred, they forged ahead. General Lane addressed the Takelmas by saying, "I promised in good faith to come into your camp, with ten unarmed men to secure peace. Myself and men are placed in your power, I do not believe that you are such cowardly dogs as to take advantage of our unarmed condition. I know that you can murder us and you can do so as quickly as you please, but what good will our blood do you? Our murder will exasperate our friends and your tribe will be hunted from the face of the earth. Let us proceed with the treaty, and in place of war, have a lasting peace." A peace treaty was signed on that day.

At the base of the Table Rock Mountains, a fort was built. Named for the general, Fort Lane consisted of a number of buildings to house Capt. A. J. Smith and his men. The men were charged with keeping the peace between the parties. All was fine in the beginning, but 1854 saw a few skirmishes. The following year peace gave way, and the Rogue Indian War was in full force. Scores of men, women, and children lost their lives on both sides. The government ordered that all Native Americans be removed to the Siletz Reservation. In October of 1856, those who had called the Rogue Valley home for generations found themselves ordered off their land and forced to march to the reservation.

One

The Early Years

James Poole and James Cluggage are credited with discovering gold during the winter of 1851–1852 in what soon became known as Table Rock City. Try as they might to keep the discovery a secret, soon they were joined by hundreds of gold miners seeking their fortunes. Some came north from California where the gold was becoming scarce, and others came south from the settlements in the Willamette Valley and as far away as Portland and Oregon City.

Those seeking their fortune staked a claim and began the backbreaking work of panning for gold during the day and sleeping wherever they could find shelter from the elements at night. Some of the men decided they could make more money hauling freight by pack-wagons than they could panning for gold. They would take their wagons, pulled by mules, to the larger settlements up north, purchase the supplies the miners needed, and then return to Jacksonville and sell the goods. Routes were established for hauling supplies to and from Crescent City where items came in on ships. Soon, a few buildings began to appear in Table Rock City and businesses opened. Families were drawn to the area, some in search of gold, others in search of land to ranch and farm. Table Rock City, named for the massive mountains off in the distance, gave way to the name of Jacksonville.

Those who settled in Jacksonville began to miss the towns they had left behind and decided their new town needed a school, a courthouse, and a church. In short order, Jacksonville began to look like the towns the pioneers had left behind.

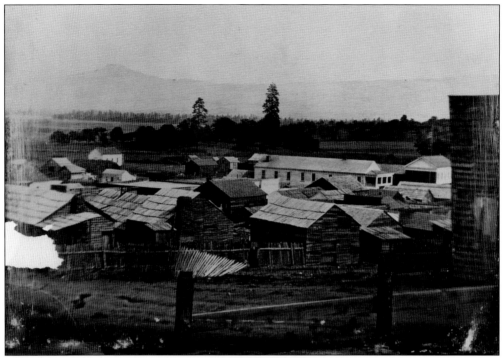

These are some of the first photographs of Jacksonville, when the town was in its infancy. In the foreground is the back of Chinatown. The photograph above was taken prior to 1854 when St. Andrew's Church was built. The photograph below shows the church as well as a few more structures.

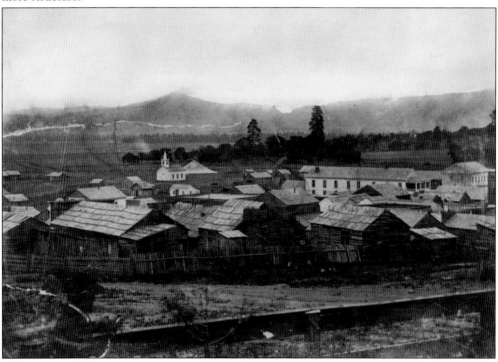

The life of a miner was not an easy one. They did not have much in the way of protective clothing, and they had to wade out in the cold streams and work hunched over for hours at a time searching for that elusive gold nugget. The gentleman shown here is crouched on a board that was placed across a small creek in Jacksonville. The miners placed their gold pan in the water hundreds of times a day, bringing it up time after time hoping to find some gold dust or a gold nugget amongst the silt and water. Some did strike it rich, but others kept moving from one area to the next. Miner Stephen Oester is pictured below with his tools. In addition to his gold pan, he has his pick and ax.

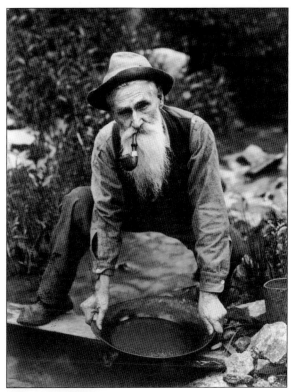

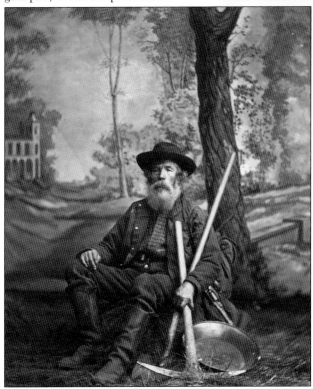

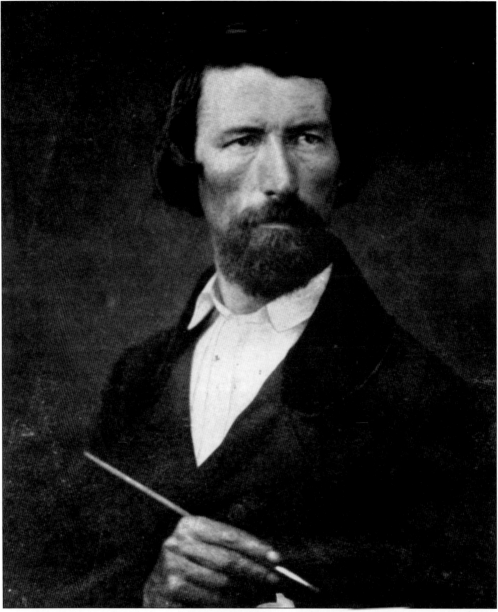

Peter Britt was born on March 19, 1819, in Obstalden, canton of Glarus, Switzerland. As a young man, he worked as a portrait and landscape painter. His work took him from one small hamlet to the next. While engaged in this line of work, he met a young lady by the name of Amalia Grob. Amalia's father did not approve of the profession that Britt had carved out for himself, and soon the relationship ended. Britt immigrated to America and settled in Illinois. He later came overland to Oregon. The years went by, but Britt always maintained contact with friends and family in Illinois. It was through such contact that he learned Amalia was living in Wisconsin with her six-year old son Jacob, and she had been recently widowed. Britt immediately wrote to her giving her two options. He offered to send her money to return to their home country or she could come to Oregon and marry him. She chose the latter and came around the Horn. They were married in a small ceremony at a friend's house. Over the years, they had three children.

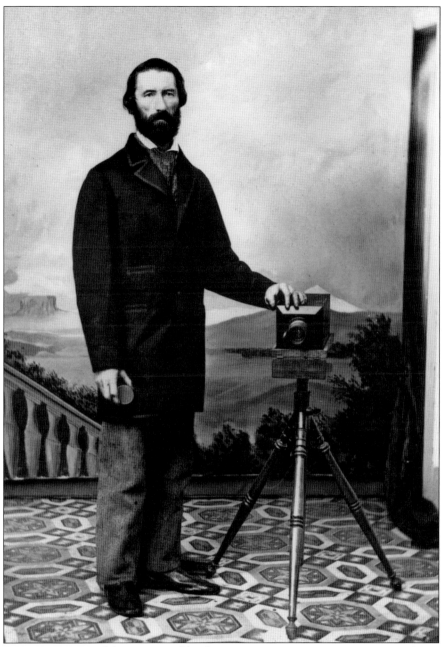

Peter Britt was a successful portrait and landscape painter prior to immigrating to America in 1845 from his home country of Switzerland. He settled in Illinois and soon learned of a new invention, the daguerreotype camera. Britt went to St. Louis and studied photography under J. H. Fitzgibbon. When he heard of the pristine new country waiting to be discovered out west, Britt decided that Oregon was the place for him to pursue a career in both painting and photography. He arrived in the Rogue Valley with $5 to his name. He tried his hand at mining for a while but soon discovered he could make more money hauling freight. He saved his money and was soon able to establish a photography and painting business in his home. Thousands of his photographs from the mid- to late-1800s have been preserved along with his photography equipment.

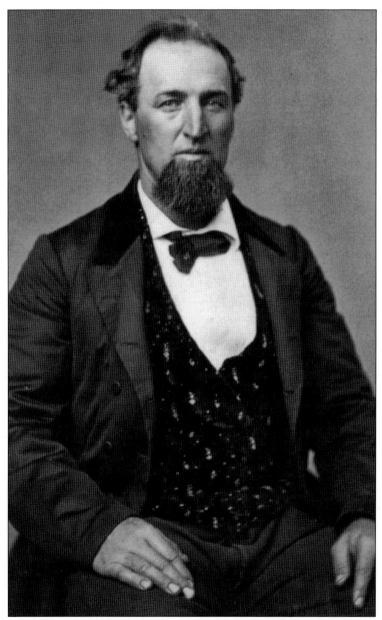

Few people left their mark on Jacksonville the way David Linn did. He began his career as a master builder, cabinetmaker, and carpenter at the age of 14. When he arrived in Jacksonville in 1853, he went right to work building sluice boxes, furniture, and basic housing for the newcomers. As time went by, he built many of the homes and churches that are still standing today. David opened a successful furniture factory. Soon after Crater Lake was discovered, David built the first boat that ever touched the lake. He built the boat in sections, then he and several other men carried the sections to the lake, put it together, and lowered it into the water. In 1863, David received a contract to build Fort Klamath. He took his sawmill by oxen team and built the fort and other buildings there. David served as Jackson County treasurer for 10 years. He traveled to Salem once a year to deliver the currency and gold to the state treasurer. For the first eight years, he made the trip on horseback.

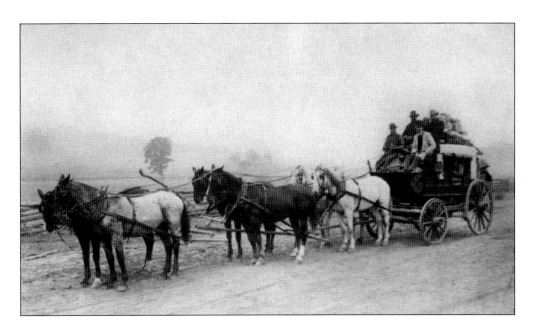

Expeditions by stagecoach were the most popular choice for traveling any distance. It was not, however, without its share of dangers. There was the possibility that the stagecoach could be held up by bandits. The stagecoach driver or "Knight of the Whip" as they were called, placed all valuables in an express box hidden under the seat. While the driver rounded curves in roads or went slowly over mountains were popular times for the bandits to venture out from their hiding spots demanding that the driver "throw down the box." Some Wells Fargo and Company stages employed an armed man to ride alongside the driver, but even that was no guarantee that the stage would not be held up. Rewards were frequently offered for the capture of the bandits but were frequently unclaimed due to the difficulty in locating a masked bandit.

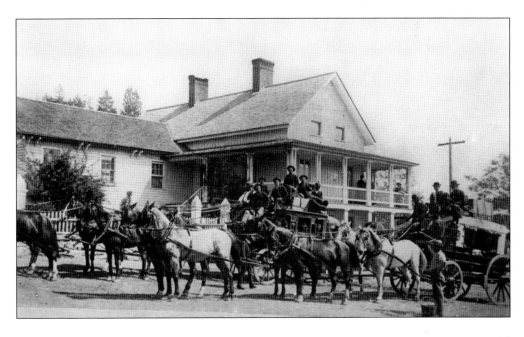

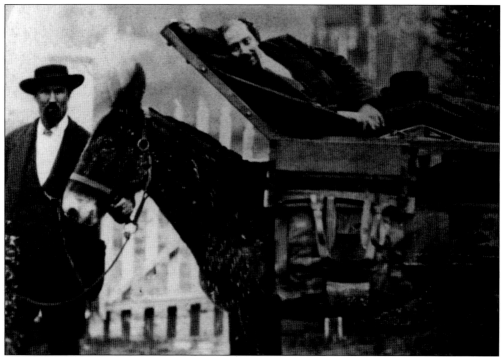

Medical science left a lot to be desired in the early days of Jacksonville. The work being done in and around Jacksonville was dangerous whether it was mining, farming, or ranching. There were many accidents, and sometimes there was no other way to get the injured to a doctor than on horseback. The photograph below shows an early day autopsy being conducted in Jacksonville.

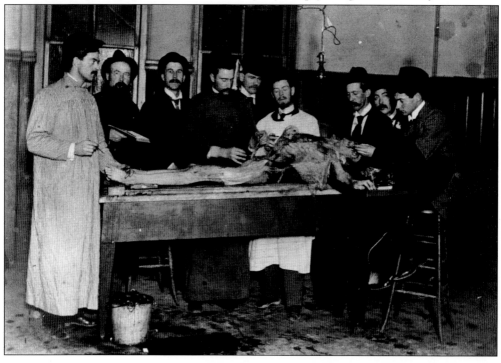

William Hoffman came overland in 1853 with his wife, Caroline, their six daughters, his two sisters, and a brother-in-law. He kept a daily journal along the way. They left Covington, Indiana, on April 13 and he wrote, "We started this day at 2 o'clock p.m. on our long journey to the Pacific Coast. The parting between our children and their juvenile friends was exceeding touching, many tears were shed. We arrived at Danville to tea, called on Brother Kingsbury and spent the night with his family." The next day he wrote, "The morning was cold with a little snow. We left our Danville friends at 8 o'clock and proceeded sixteen miles to feed." On July 1 he wrote, "At 10 o'clock we arrived at the upper end of the valley at Scotts Bluff. Here the scenery is unsurpassed. It is worth a great deal of toil to witness so beautiful a picture." Upon arriving in the Rogue Valley he wrote, "We have been to Jacksonville twice and examined a number of (donation) claims from which we have made no selection yet."

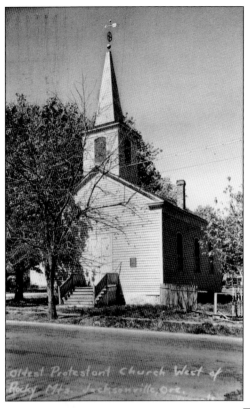

In 1852, William Kahler arrived in Jacksonville with his wife and six children. Kahler donated money and sold his last yoke of oxen, valued at $150, so that a church could be built in Jacksonville. The church still stands today, and is known as St. Andrew's Anglican Church. Rev. Thomas F. Royal spent many years as a circuit rider traveling from one town to another helping to build churches including St. Andrew's. He used his saddlebags to carry his religious materials, clothing, food for himself, and oats for his horse. He spoke of the saddlebags saying, "These I know look old and wrinkled enough to have seen a century's use. If you would like to know where the wrinkles came from, ask the stormy winds and pelting rains. Ask the black splattering mud of southern Oregon."

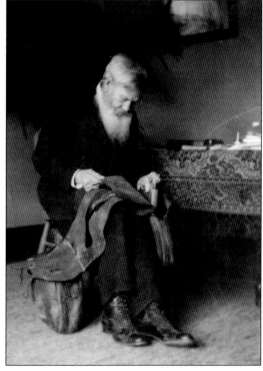

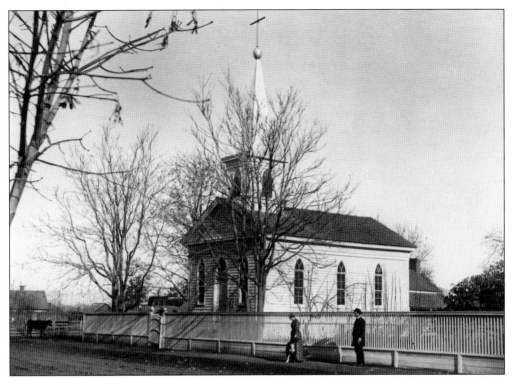

St. Joseph's Catholic Church was dedicated in November 1858. The bell that beckoned the townsfolk to Sunday mass weighed 297 pounds and was cast in Sheffield, England, and then shipped around the Horn. Father Blanchet arrived in Jacksonville in 1864 and took over as the priest. He recalled traveling by carriage 150 miles round-trip in the pouring rain to visit a man who was dying of consumption. Father Blanchet spent 25 years as the priest of St. Joseph's. At one time, he returned to his native Montreal for a short while and wrote a book, *Ten Years on the Pacific Coast*. In 1875, Father Blanchet purchased the small white cottage just down the street from the church. He lived there until 1888 when he was named pastor of a Catholic church in St. Paul, Oregon.

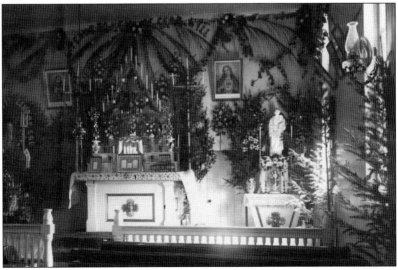

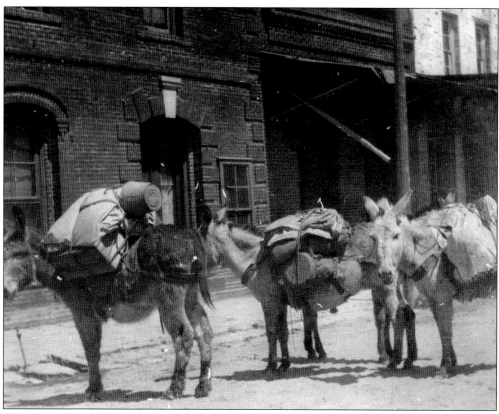

The pack mules shown here are ready for another day of work hauling supplies. They are in front of the Brunner building on Oregon Street. Mules proved their worth by being able to carry heavy goods to and from Jacksonville. They had no problems with the terrain and were able to make it through the brush where wagons could not go. In the photograph below, the dog is proving that although he may not be helping to haul any supplies, he is still "Man's best friend."

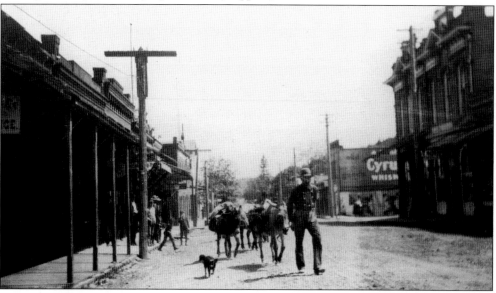

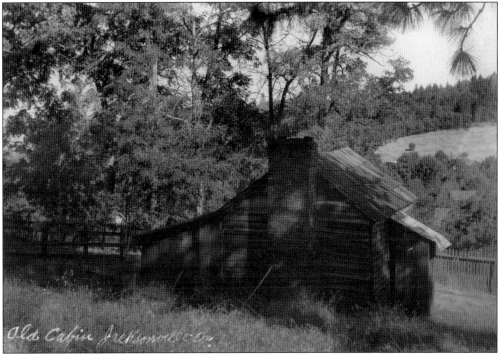

Whether they traveled by sea or came across the plains, it was imperative that the pioneers arrived prior to the first cold weather in Oregon. The trip overland took approximately six months, so the pioneers left from "jump off" points in Missouri by early spring. Once they arrived at their destination, they had to get their shelter built and their crops in before winter came. These photographs show a basic cabin that would have sheltered the family until they had the means to build something more substantial.

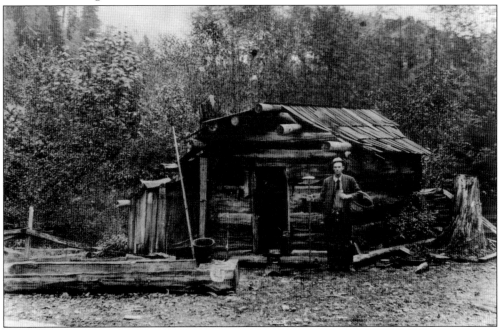

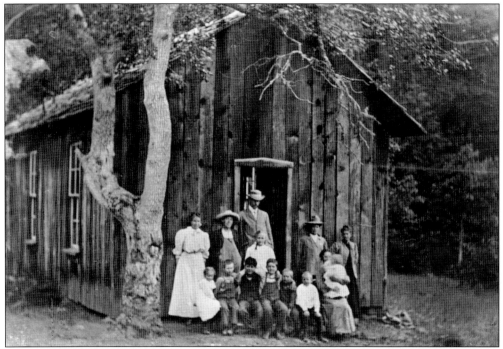

Even a small cabin could be home to many family members, as pictured above. There was no electricity or indoor plumbing, so things were rather primitive. In Jacksonville, most families used kerosene lanterns for their source of light. In the evenings, the families would read, play games, write letters back home, and help the children with their studies. The cabin below has a nice front porch where the family could spend many summer evenings.

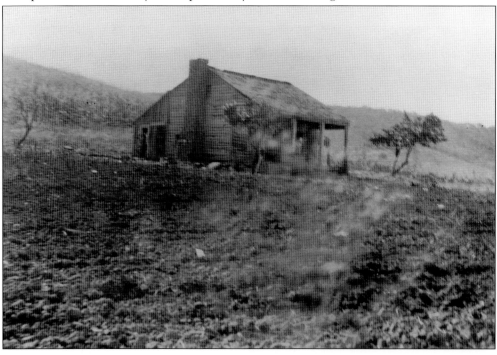

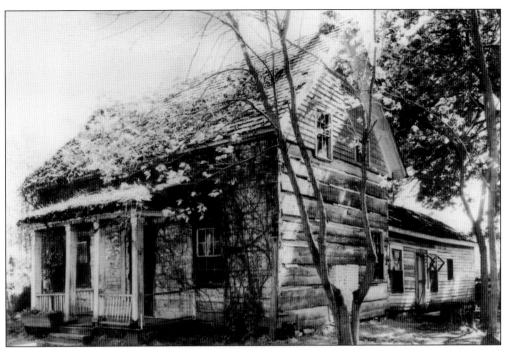

Once the pioneers decided to stay in a particular area, it was not uncommon to add onto their cabin. The house above not only has an addition, but it also has windows. The foundation is mainly wood and rocks. Other settlers abandoned their cabin for a brand new house, as pictured below.

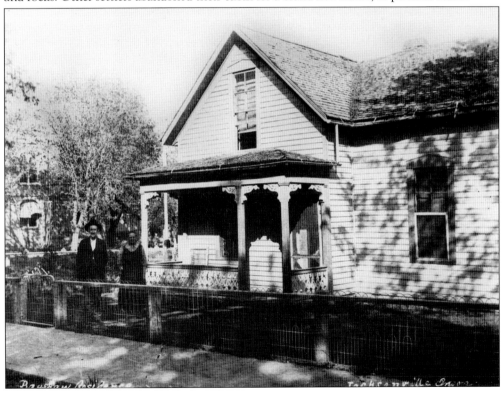

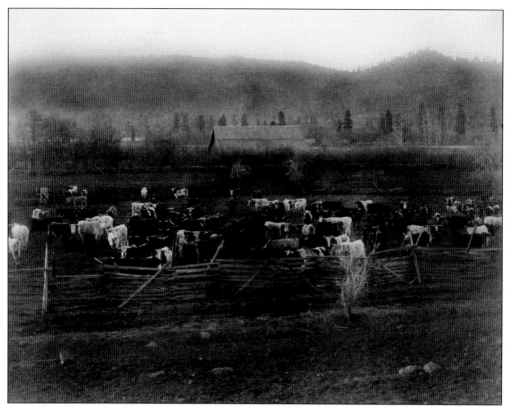

Many of Jacksonville's first farmers raised stock. The meat was in great demand and the hides were put to use as well. David Linn used the hides for seats in the chairs that he made. John Orth ran a butcher shop from his building on Oregon Street. This photograph below, taken by Peter Britt, gives new meaning to the expression, "When the cows come home," as they seem to have done just that.

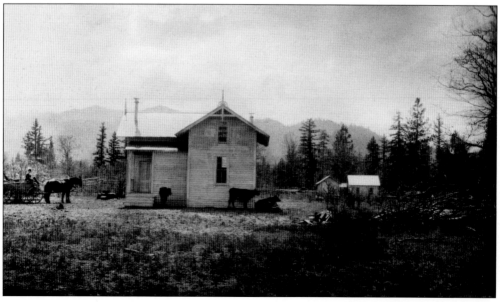

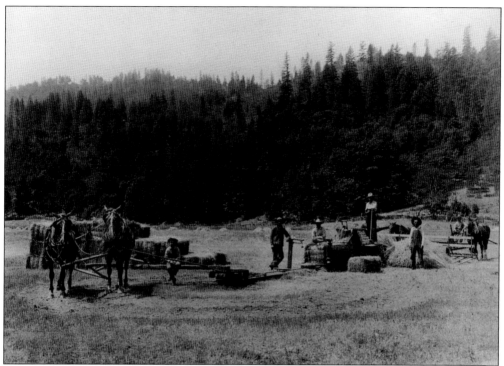

Many of the early settlers took Donation Land Claims and began farming the land. Growing hay was a common vocation in Jacksonville. Pictured above, the men are baling the hay and preparing it for market. The farmers only had very basic equipment and everything was done by hand. It was common for school-age boys to work through the harvest helping their fathers and then begin school after the harvest. This team of horses is pulling a wagon filled with hay. Today technology has created machines to do much of the work that farm animals used to do.

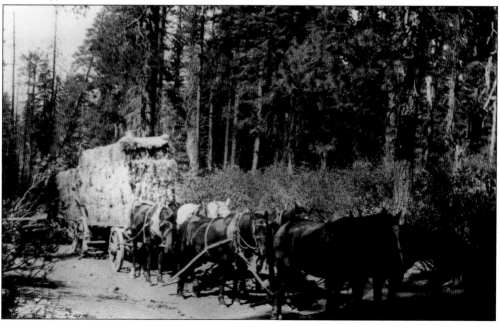

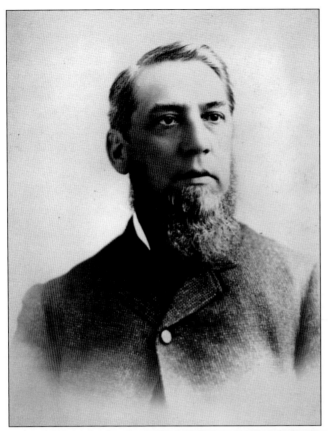

Cornelius C. Beekman was born and raised in Dundee, New York. At the age of 22, he struck out for the west by way of the isthmus of Panama. He did some mining and carpentry work in California, then he began carrying express between Yreka and Jacksonville. In 1863, he opened a bank in Jacksonville. It was the first bank in southern Oregon and the second bank in Oregon. If someone needed a loan, Cornelius would loan his own money, but he never risked the bank's money. Instead of paying people interest on their money, he charged people for storing their money. When a customer wanted to make a withdrawal or a deposit, Cornelius handed them their own pouch where their money was stored. Today Beekman Bank is exactly as it was in 1915, the last time it was open.

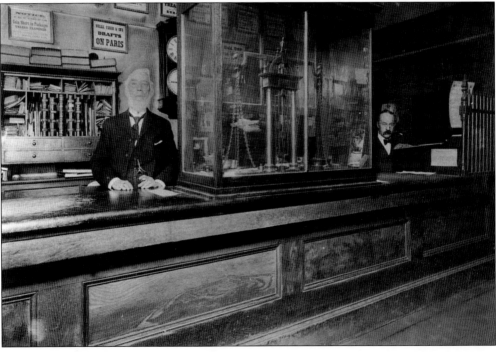

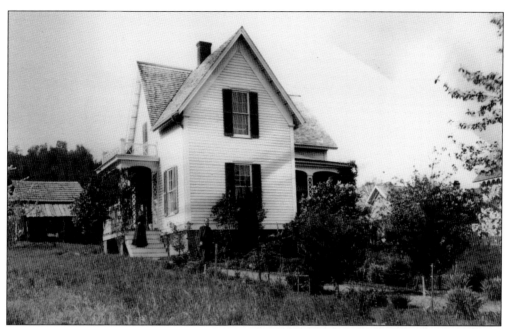

Cornelius and Julia Beekman are pictured here in front of their home. Beekman may very well be heading off to work at his bank. The Beekmans were married in 1861 and moved into a small house on the corner of California and Sixth Streets that still stands today. Their three children, Benjamin, Carrie, and Lydia, were born there. In the mid-1870s, the family had this house built. They were the only people who ever lived in the house. They received electricity in 1905 that replaced their kerosene lanterns. In 1915, the Beekmans had indoor plumbing installed. The interior of the house and all of the furnishings remain just as they were in the year 1911. The kitchen is pictured below complete with the woodstove they purchased in 1904 from Kenney's hardware store in Jacksonville.

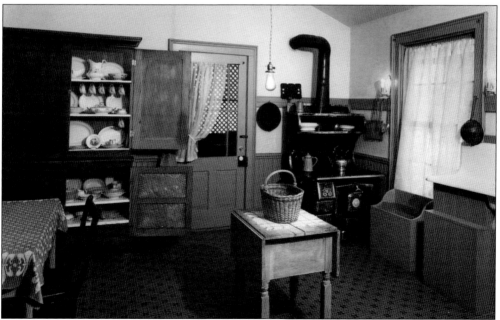

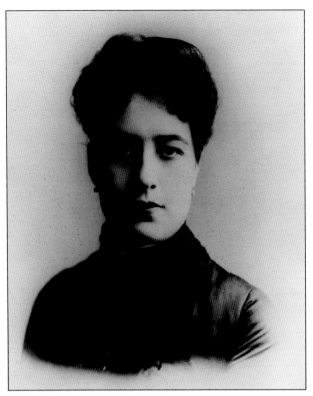

Carrie Beekman grew up in Jacksonville and attended Mills Seminary (later renamed Mills College) near Oakland, California. Once she finished her studies at Mills Seminary, she returned to Jacksonville, taught Sunday school at the Presbyterian church, and gave piano lessons to many young girls in town. She traveled a great deal; the highlight of her travels was when she joined her cousin Ruth on an 18-month journey to Ireland, England, and throughout much of Europe. Carrie looked after her parents as they got on in years. She was the last surviving member of the family. When she died in 1959, she bequeathed the house, bank, and all of the furnishings to the University of Oregon. Jackson County currently owns the properties.

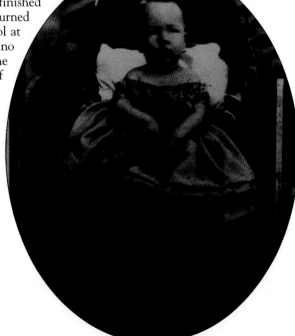

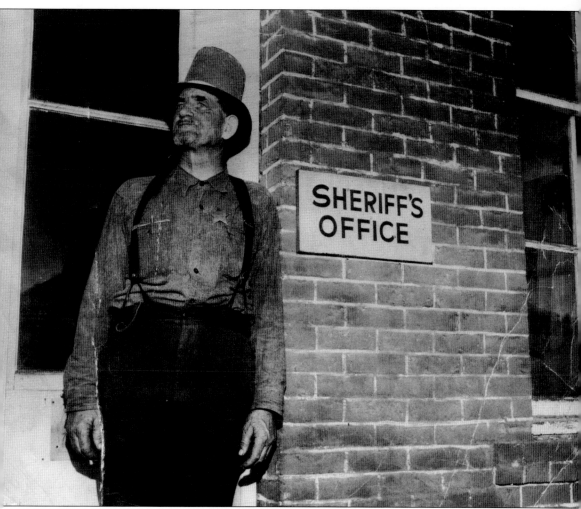

Sheriff Isaac Coffman is pictured here outside of the Jacksonville jail. It would seem that there was not much time to be standing around based on a newspaper article from 1866 that read: "Juvenile depravity seems to be on the increase. There is a crowd of boys ages 8 to fifteen that can swear with great volubility and seem to want only a few more years of street education to qualify them for the penitentiary or the gallows." An article from 1868 stated, "Burglars About! Some scoundrels broke into the home of old Mrs. Bellinger and took away quite a number of articles of wearing apparel. After ransacking the old lady's trunk, the scamps deliberately went to work and cooked supper. We advise our citizens to be on the lookout and keep a shotgun handy for nocturnal thieves."

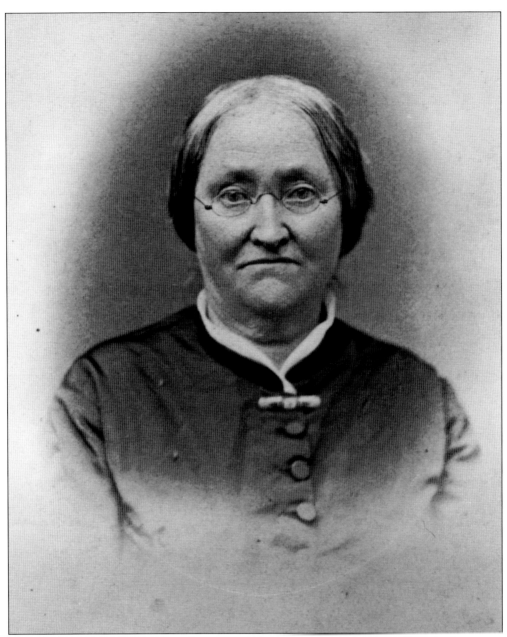

During the summer of 1861, political tensions were running deep in Jacksonville and other towns across the country. One morning, the locals discovered that someone had run a Confederate flag up the flagpole on California Street right in the center of town. "Aunty" Zany Ganung, wife of Dr. Louis Ganung, noticed not only the flag but also that none of the men standing around watching it sway in the breeze were doing anything about it. Determined to not let this emblem belittle the country she believed in, legend has it that she armed herself with a gun and an ax and headed out the front door of her house. She approached the flagpole, placed the gun on the ground, and proceeded to swing the ax until the entire flagpole came crashing down. She picked up her weapon and the offending flag and returned home. Soon after, smoke could be seen coming from her chimney.

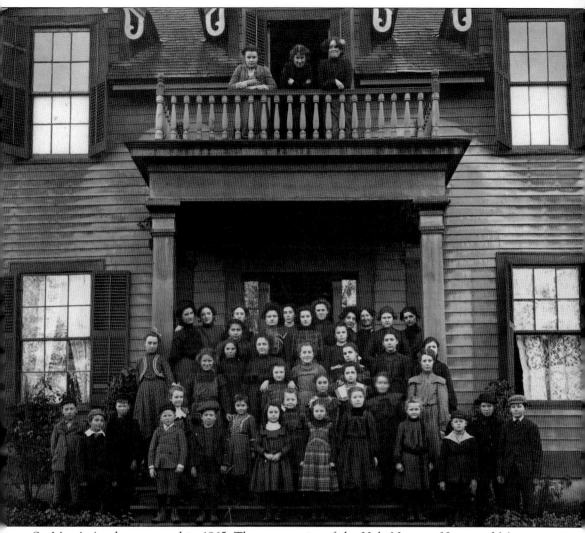

St. Mary's Academy opened in 1865. The community of the Holy Names of Jesus and Mary agreed to open a school in Jacksonville at Father Blanchet's request. Three sisters spent months traveling by boat from Montreal to Portland, then by carriage from Portland to Jacksonville, to teach the students. The academy taught local children as well as children who were from out of the area and lived at the academy during the school year.

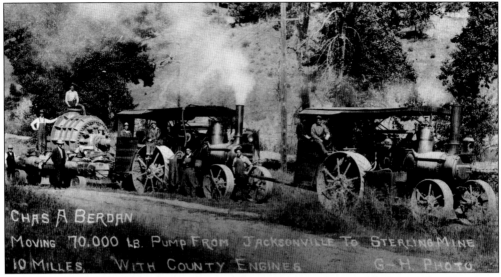

CHAS A BERDAN
MOVING 70,000 LB. PUMP FROM JACKSONVILLE TO STERLING MINE
10 MILLES, WITH COUNTY ENGINES   G-H. PHOTO

Once the easy gold had been panned out of the creeks in and around Jacksonville, the miners began looking for other ways to extract the hidden gold. It was decided that hydraulic mining was the way to go, but bringing the necessary equipment to the area was no easy feat as shown in the picture above. To operate the machinery, workers diverted water from nearby ditches into a penstock made from riveted steel pipe. The penstock ran downhill and the water was discharged into a large iron muzzle, known as a "giant." The giant blasted the sides of the hill with tremendous force, thereby loosening the soil. The soil was washed through sluice boxes that trapped the gold dust and nuggets. Hydraulic mining was banned in the area by the late 1800s due to the damage to the land.

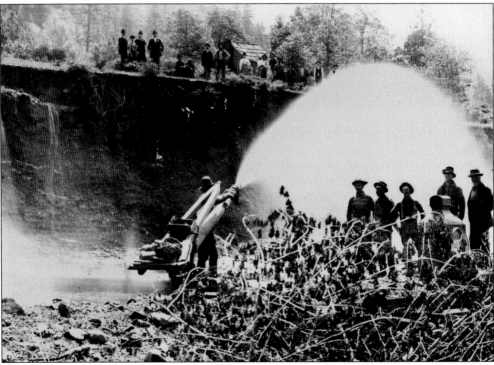

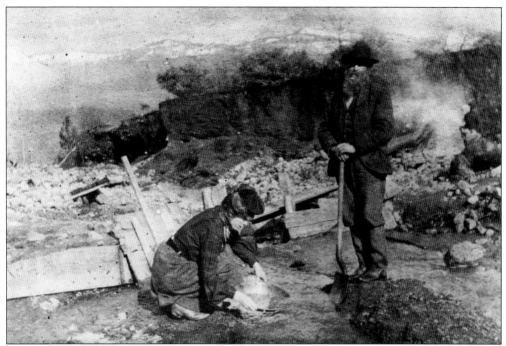

In an obvious role reversal, the female shown here is demonstrating to the male just how to pan for gold. In the photograph below, everyone seems a bit puzzled by the female who is helping with the operation.

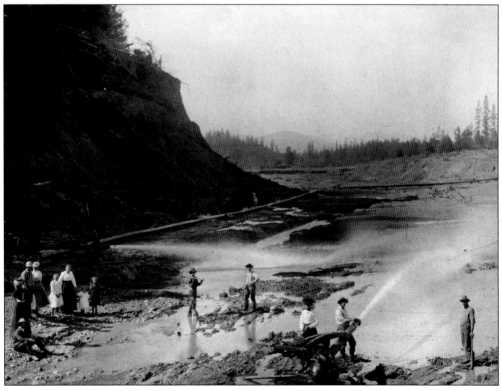

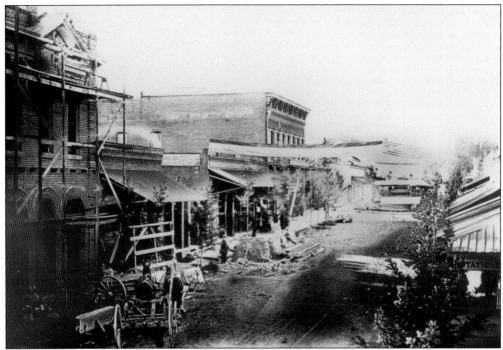

Following two devastating fires that swept through downtown Jacksonville, the business owners decided it would be best to use bricks for all future construction. That proved to be a good idea as many of the brick buildings are still standing today. However, it was very time-consuming because the bricks were made just outside of Jacksonville using local materials, then hauled into town. Each building was then built by hand using the local bricks. The Jacksonville Brick and Tile Company is pictured below.

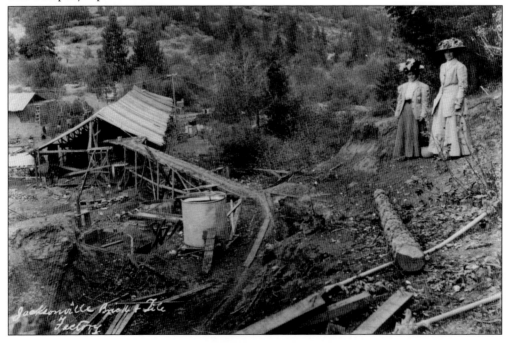

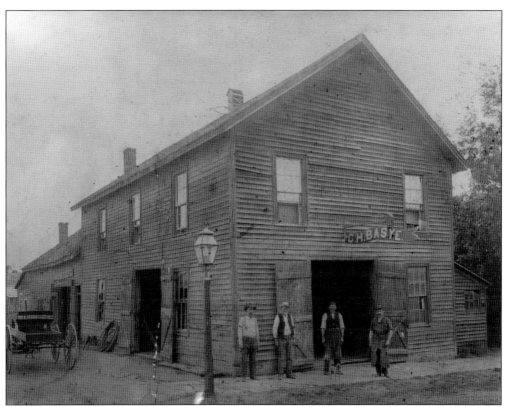

There was a time when downtown Jacksonville had three blacksmith shops, all of which were very busy. The locals would stop in for a chat and watch the men do their work. The blacksmiths stayed busy repairing wagon wheels, fixing buggies, shoeing horses, and sharpening tools used for gold mining such as drill picks and plow shears. Charles Bayse (who later became a jailor and was killed during a jail break) is pictured above, at far right, in front of his blacksmith shop. He made shackles, balls, and chains for the prisoners of the jail.

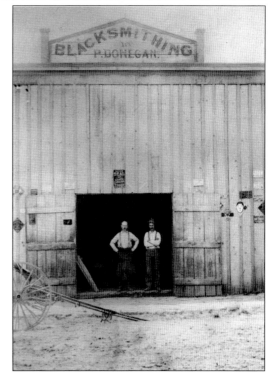

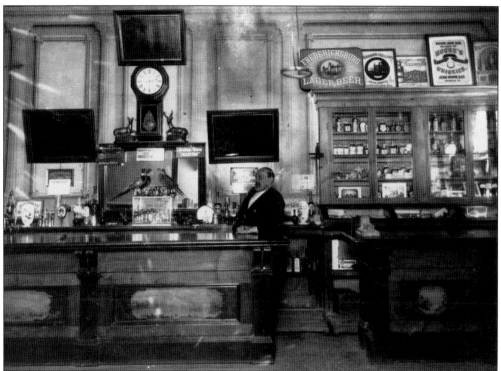

Herman Von Helms immigrated to America from Holstein, Germany, at the age of 21. As soon as he arrived in Jacksonville, he took a look around and decided the town needed a bakery. Herman and his partner, John Wintjen, opened one. Next they opened the Table Rock Saloon. They sent for a billiard table, which came around the Horn to Crescent City and was packed in by freight wagons pulled by mules. The Table Rock Saloon went on to become one of Jacksonville's longest running businesses. Herman's oldest son, Ed, took over the operation and ran it until his own retirement in 1914. Herman asked the locals to share items from the Takelma Indians, minerals and rocks, freaks of nature, coins, and other oddities for what became Jacksonville's first museum, as pictured below.

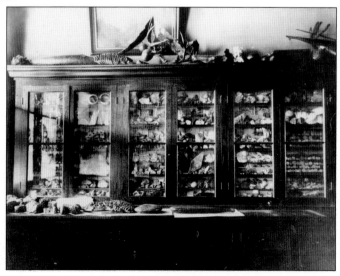

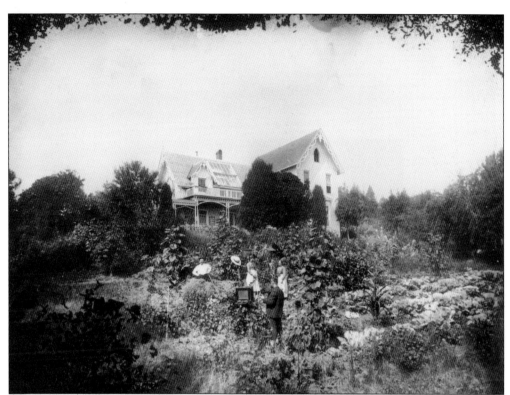

In addition to his painting and photography work, Peter Britt became a great horticulturist. He created a beautiful park-like setting on his property. There were already wild grapes growing in the area, but Britt brought cuttings from established mission vines in California and soon he had the first vineyard in the area. He devoted 15 acres to grapes and began bottling wine under the name of Valley View Vineyards. In 1857, Britt purchased some fruit cuttings from a peddler who had arrived from California. In short order, Britt was growing apples, pears, and peaches. The locals were astonished when they saw the exotic plants Britt was growing such as a palm tree, an Abyssinian banana tree, cactus, kumquats, lemons, oranges, coffee bushes, figs, pomegranates, rhododendrons, and wisteria and magnolia trees.

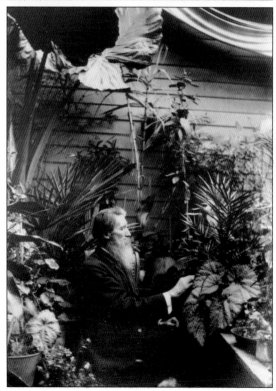

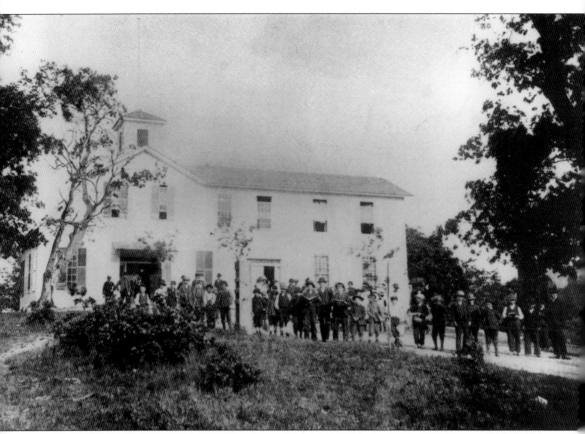
The first schoolhouse in Jacksonville was established in 1854. It was a single-room cabin on Old Stage Road. In 1866, the School District Trustees raised enough money to build a new schoolhouse on Bigham Knoll. The students pictured here are standing in front of their new school in 1868. The tuition was $5 per quarter and there were two quarters in a school year.

During the small pox epidemic of 1868, four Catholic nuns in Jacksonville ran a "pest house" for those infected with the dreaded disease. The sick would be brought to the pest house and the nuns would care for them round the clock. No one was allowed to visit. If the person stricken with small pox succumbed to the illness, then Father Blanchet helped bury them. Fear of catching the disease kept friends and family from attending the funeral. The funerals were sometimes held under the cover of darkness in the Jacksonville cemetery. During this time, the locals believed they could kill the germs with smoke, so they burned pitch pine in the streets day and night. After two months, the small pox epidemic was over, but many people lost their lives in northern California and southern Oregon.

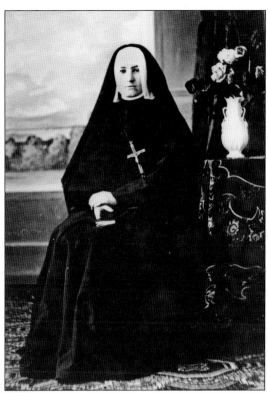

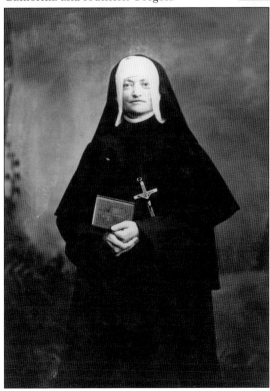

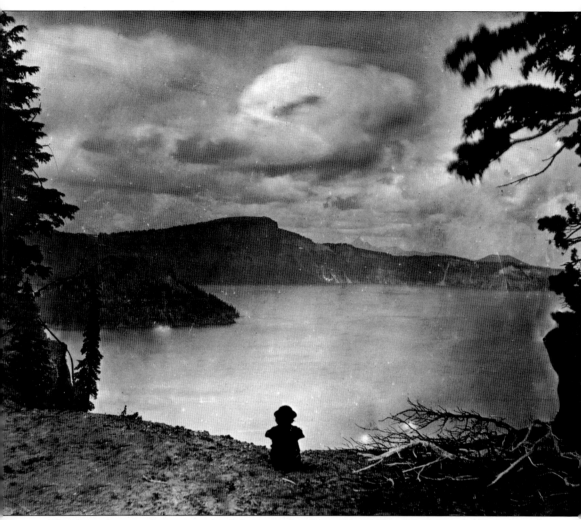

The first white settlers to see this lake named it Deep Blue Lake. The lake was later named Crater Lake. Peter Britt is credited with taking the first photograph of it. In 1874, he set out from his home with 200 pounds of photography equipment in his wagon. He was accompanied by his 12-year-old son, Emil, and two other men. It took five days for them to reach the lake. In order to photograph it, Peter needed sunlight and the weather was not cooperating. Finally, after two days of fog and mist, the skies brightened and Peter was able to capture the first photographs of Crater Lake. His diary for Thursday, August 13, 1874, simply read, "Photographed the lake. Very cold and windy. Emil had a cough."

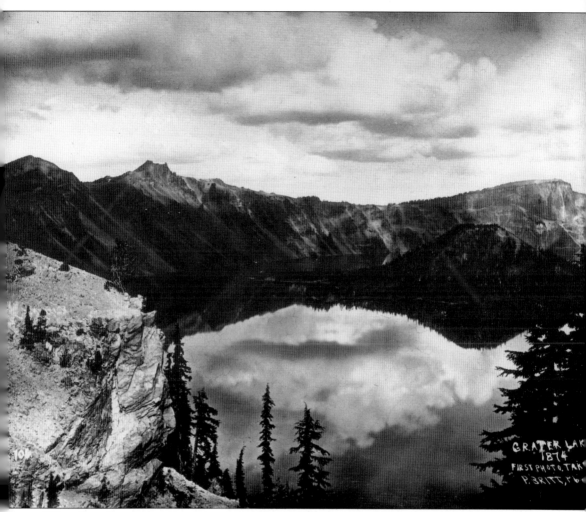

When Peter Britt was ready to photograph Crater Lake, he set up his black tent, quickly coated his glass plate negatives with a liquid chemical, and then took two, 20-second exposure images. He remained under his black tent for approximately 30 minutes before emerging with 2 negatives that were completely developed. The photographs he took on August 13, 1874, were the first images of the lake. During the 17 years that William Gladstone Steel fought to have Crater Lake declared a national park, he used the photographs taken by Peter in 1874 to convince others the area should be preserved. Finally, in 1902, Congress approved the bill naming Crater Lake a national park.

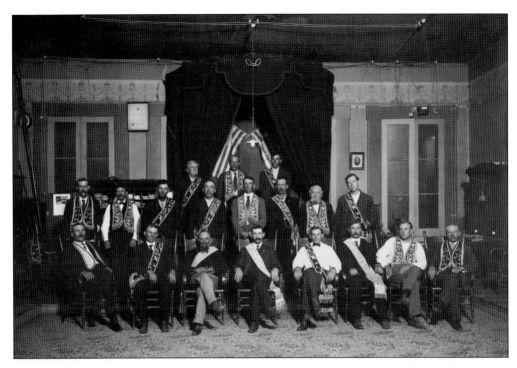

The Independent Order of Odd Fellow Lodge No. 10 in Jacksonville was established on June 30, 1860. The main concern of this fraternal organization was the welfare of the brethren. They looked after one another and came to each other's aid if someone was experiencing difficult times. The Odd Fellows allowed the Jewish citizens the use of their lodge on their holy days. Their lodge stands today on Main and Oregon Streets. The men are pictured in their regalia while inside the lodge. Below is a picture that includes the women of the Rebekah Lodge, a group for women.

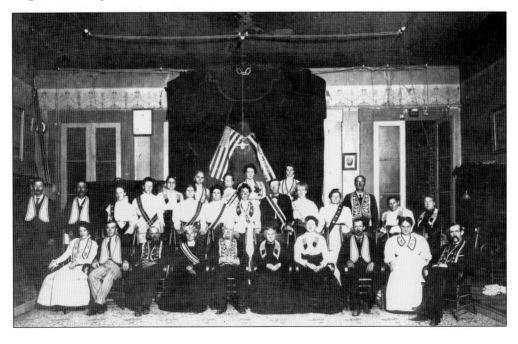

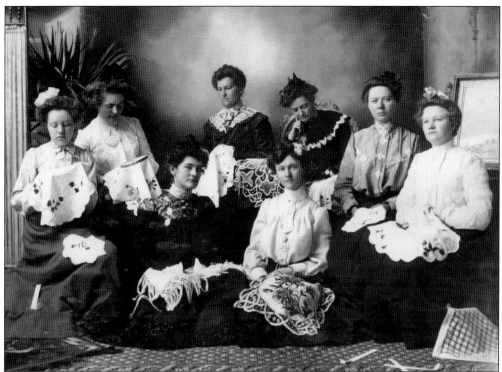

The women pictured here are taking a well deserved break. Pioneer women raised the children, kept the house, did the cooking and baking, chopped wood for the cook stove, hauled water in and out of the house for washing and bathing, washed and ironed the clothing, sewed and mended the family's clothing, went into town to purchase food and essentials, helped feed the farm animals and the chickens or turkeys, gathered eggs, churned butter, and milked cows.

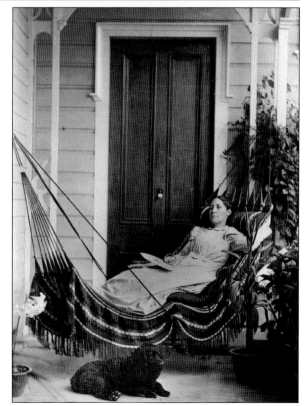

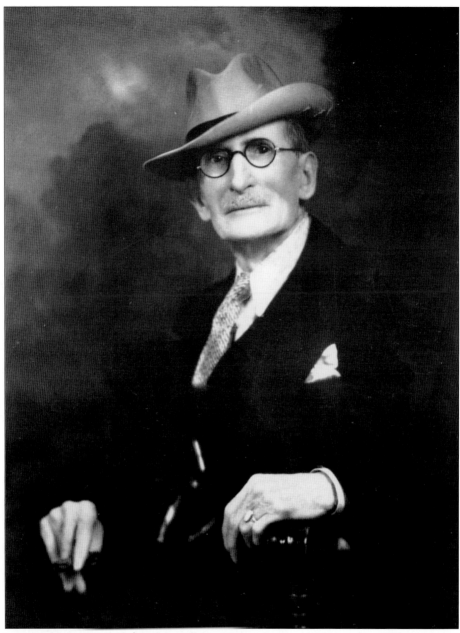

Dr. James Robinson arrived in Jacksonville in 1878 and was quoted as saying, "When I arrived in this beautiful valley, which was on a Sunday evening I felt I had found my paradise. The church bells were ringing as I entered the old mining town of Jacksonville and these musical tones seemed to be a welcome." Life in Jacksonville would not be easy for Dr. Robinson though. His wife, Ella, one of the first physicians in Oregon, died less than a year after they opened a practice together in Jacksonville. A few years later, he married Matilda (Tillie) Miller and they had two children, a boy named Willie Cecil, and a girl named Mary Leah. The children died from diphtheria within days of each other when they were five and six years old. Referring to his life as a physician, Dr. Robinson said, "My work was hard, the roads were bad and many times I made rides of 50 miles one way, 100 miles round trip when the rain was pouring and the wind was blowing."

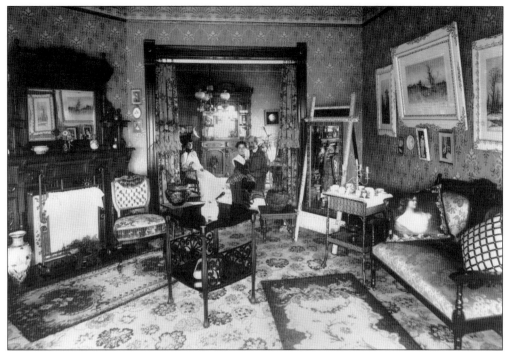

A few years later, the Robinsons had a little girl they named Regina Dorland. Dorland, as she was called, grew up to be a gifted artist. She is seen here with her parents inside their home and doing some painting near the pond at Peter Britt's house. Dorland studied art back east as well as in the Bay Area of California under some of the best teachers. Her parents accompanied her on these trips and shielded her from much of the outside world. By the time she was in her early twenties, she was becoming a well-known artist. While studying art in California, she met a young man and they married soon after. The marriage did not last and for reasons that remain unknown, Dorland tragically took her own life shortly after the divorce at the age of 26.

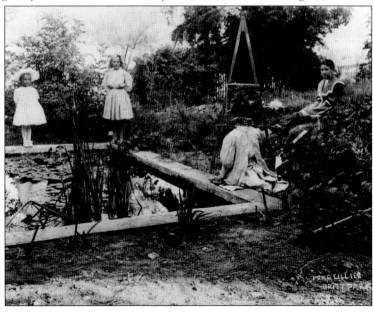

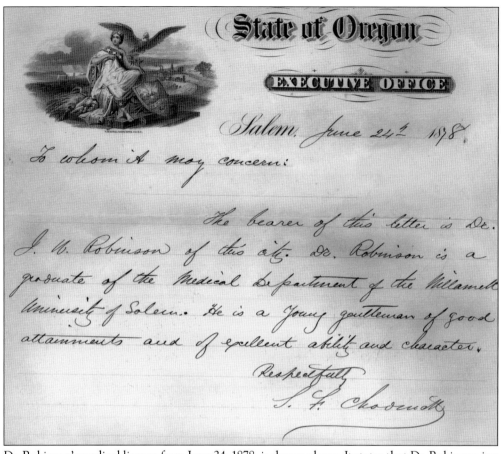

Dr. Robinson's medical license from June 24, 1878, is shown above. It states that Dr. Robinson is a graduate of the Medical Department of the Willamette University of Salem. It goes on to say that, "He is a young gentleman of good attainments and of excellent ability and character." The receipt below shows the prices Dr. Robinson charged for his medical services in Jacksonville. A daytime visit in town was $3, a night visit in town was $4, obstetrics were $20, and all services cost an extra $5 if you lived in the country. This receipt indicates Dr. Robinson's client had run up a tab of $10 but had paid him with 2 chickens and 23 pounds of lard, thus reducing his bill to $6.

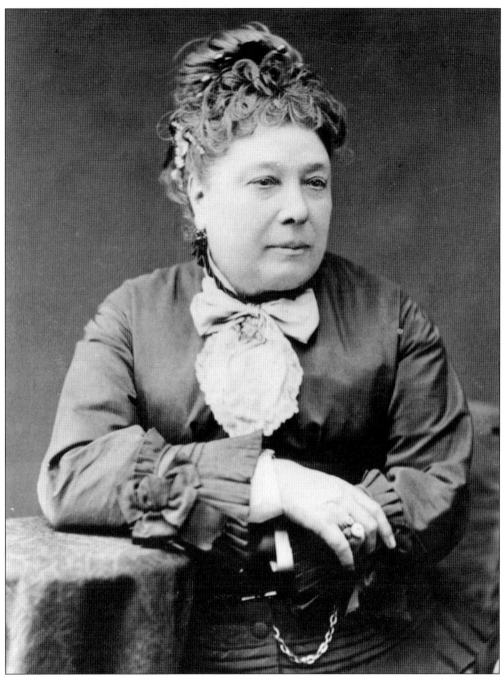

Jeane De Roboam was originally from Bordeaux, France. She ran the Franco-American hotel in Jacksonville. Her hotel was near the stage stop in Jacksonville, and many a weary passenger took refuge there. The locals referred to her as Madame DeRoboam. Jeane was no wallflower and was known for her exuberance of life. She married George Holt, one of Jacksonville's finest bricklayers. Soon George found himself building her a new two-story hotel made from brick, which they named the U.S. Hotel.

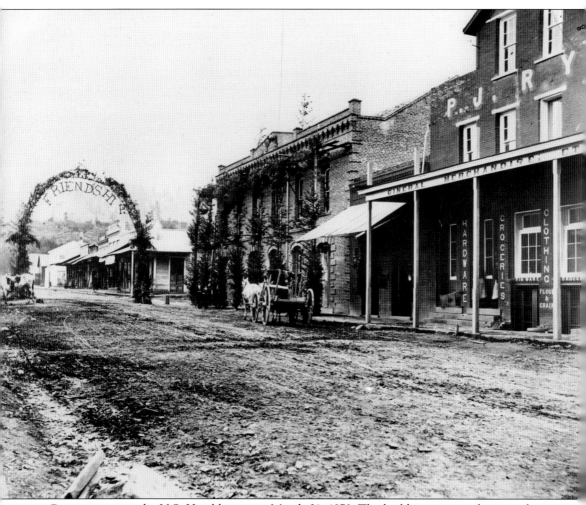

Construction on the U.S. Hotel began on March 21, 1879. The building was not done yet, but that did not stop the locals from having a grand ball on the Fourth of July that year. Two months later, the hotel was still not done when word was received that President Hayes, his wife Lucy, Gen. William T. Sherman, and the president's physician and his wife would be traveling through Jacksonville and would need overnight accommodations. Legend has it that the next morning Madame Holt presented her bill to General Sherman. He was shocked at the amount for a one-night stay. He is said to have pointed out to Madame Holt that the Palace Hotel in San Francisco was only $6 per night. When this failed to change her mind, it has been said that General Sherman told her he did not wish to purchase the hotel but merely to pay for a night's stay. Legend has it that Madame Holt got her asking price.

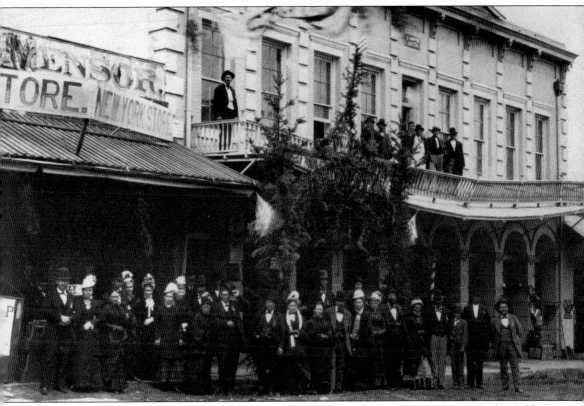

Jacksonville had many fraternal organizations in the early days such as the Masons, the Odd Fellows, and the Order of the Redman, which was reserved for those of German descent. In this photograph from 1880, men and women have traveled from Yreka, California, and Linkville (known today as Klamath Falls) to celebrate St. Tammany's Day. The men on the balcony do not seem at all concerned about their precarious situation.

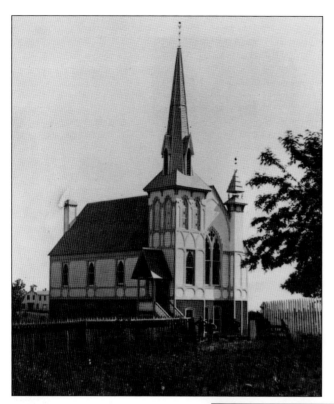

The Presbyterian Church in Jacksonville is one of the most beautiful churches in the valley. It was built by David Linn and dedicated in 1881. The stained glass windows were shipped around the Horn from Italy and then packed in wagons led by mules. The town banker, Cornelius Beekman, donated a substantial portion of the funds needed. Other money was raised by strawberry, lemonade, and ice cream socials and other fundraising events to raise the $6,000 needed to build the church. Fr. Moses Williams was the minister. In his diaries, he wrote, "When I wish to read my Bible, there is no light scarcely in the house from the want of windows. When it is not too cold the doors are set open for light." The lads pictured below are from a Sunday school class.

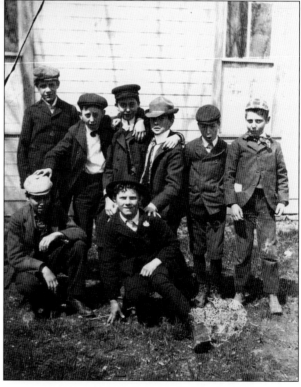

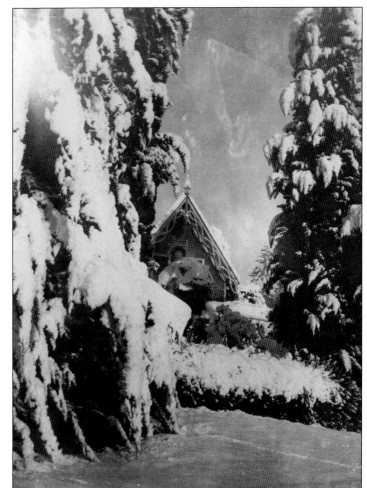

The winters in Jacksonville could be very harsh, as pictured here. The Britt home is covered with snow, making it look like a winter wonderland. The children pictured below are enjoying a day off from school or chores. The Von Helms house is on the left and the Britt home is at the top of the hill.

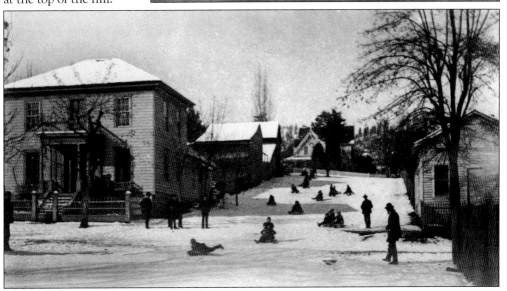

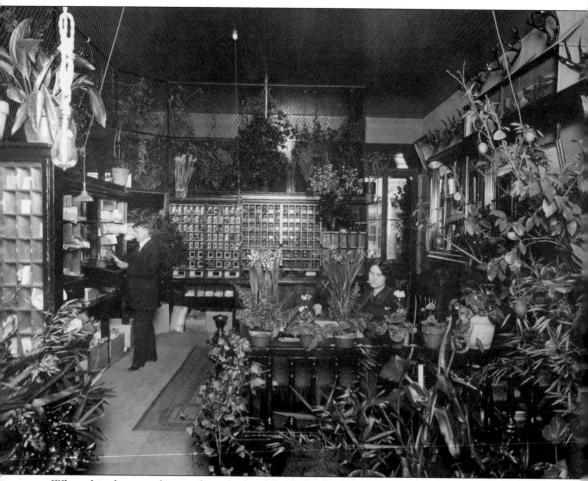

When this photograph was taken, the locals had to collect their mail at the post office. Even today, the United States Post Office has a limited delivery schedule for the residents of Jacksonville. When the locals walk into the post office these days, they are not greeted with such fine greenery. The interior greenery shown here appears to be the handiwork of Peter Britt.

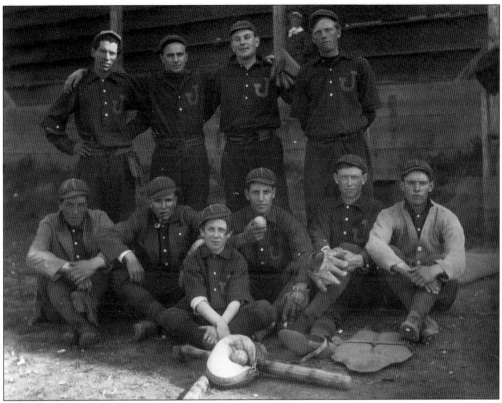

The Jacksonville baseball team used to play against teams in Ashland and Gold Hill. The boys would travel in freight wagons pulled by horses. It took several hours each way to reach Ashland or Gold Hill. Pictured above in the front row, from left to right, are Ike Dundford, Gordon Stout, Bill McIntyre, Ed Wendt, and Curly Wilson. In the second row are Pat Donagon, Ray Sexton, Leslie Ulrich, and Charley Dundford. The team mascot, Hal Hines, is seated in front.

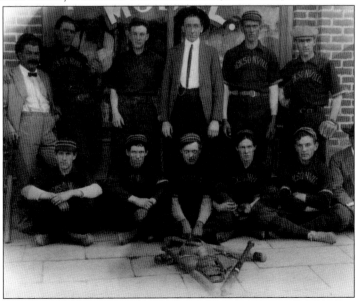

53

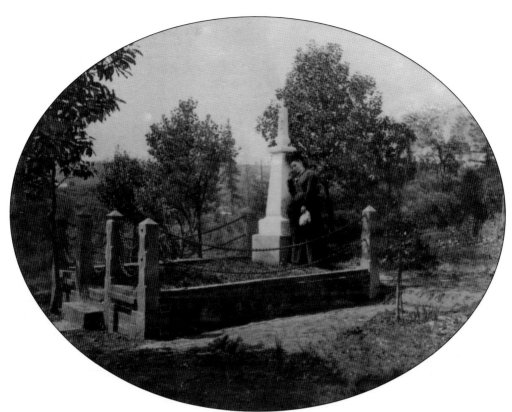

During the Victorian Era in Jacksonville, as well as in other towns across the country, women practiced certain customs. The customs originated in England. If a woman's husband died, she was expected to maintain the Victorian mourning customs as much as possible. There were three phases of mourning. During the first phase, women could only wear black dresses made from crepe material that had no sheen to them. The second phase allowed her to wear gray, and finally the third phase allowed for some violet. The entire process varied from area to area, but it could be for an entire year. During that time, her social activities were curtailed and she was not allowed to remarry. If a man's wife died, he was expected to wear a black band around his arm for three months and after that time he could remarry.

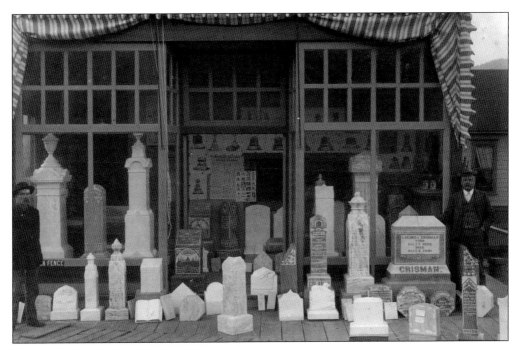

The Marble Works business located on the corner of California and Oregon Streets provided the locals with a place to choose a monument for their loved one when the time came. Prior to the establishment of this business, locals had to order a monument from back east and have it shipped around the Horn. During the late 1800s, it was believed that the fancier the monument, the better. It was not only a sign of your wealth, but also a sign of respect for your loved one. The Bybee monument below shows a family monument as well as individual monuments.

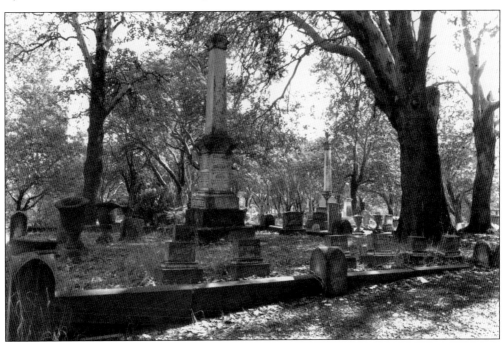

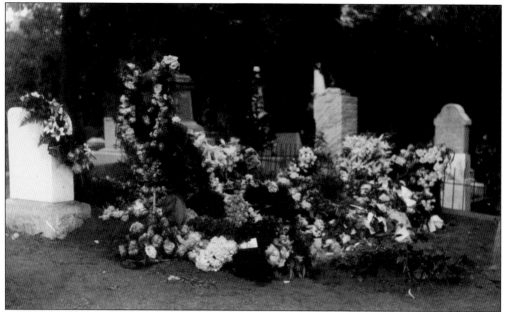

During the late 1800s, there were certain customs that a family took part in when a loved one died. First, you would cover your front door with black crepe material. You would stop all the clocks in the house until after the funeral. You would turn all mirrors towards the walls. You would send out death notices to family and friends. If you received a death notice, you were expected to attend the funeral unless you were pregnant. There were no funeral homes in those days, so the body of the loved one laid in rest in the parlor of the family home until the church service and burial. At the gravesite, family and friends left flowers as pictured here for Theodoric (Todd) Cameron and Mary Day.

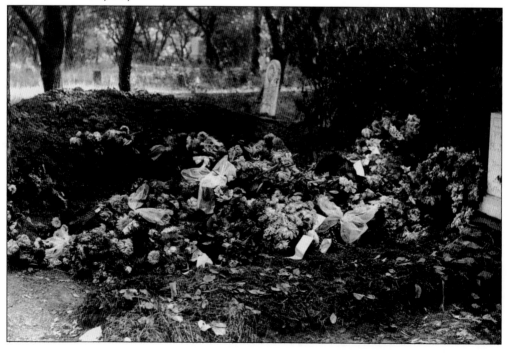

Two
The Chinese and Other Minorities

They were called Celestials or Sojourners, but neither term was spoken in a positive manner. They were the Chinese who had traveled so far, not to begin a new life here, but instead to work hard to earn money so when they returned home they would be better off financially. The journey was long and difficult in cramped quarters, and once on American soil they were met by a "China boss" who took them to their new job. They were already in debt to their new boss for the passage to America and for the food they had consumed on the ship. They had no choice but to work hard to pay him back. Those that arrived in Table Rock City established their own Chinatown. The houses were constructed from whatever materials they could obtain and they crowded into their new homes. The Chinese honored their customs and kept to themselves. Many of the white settlers ridiculed them because of their customs. The Chinese had a firm belief that if you died in a foreign country, your body would not be at rest if it was not returned to China. When a Chinese person died in Jacksonville, their body was buried in the Jacksonville Cemetery in an elaborate ceremony. As the body was brought up the hill to the cemetery, the Chinese would toss slips of fake money onto the ground with the name of the deceased. Once at the grave, they set out a feast of food including roast pork. They brought clothing of the deceased and laid it on the grave. It was their belief that in providing the deceased with money, food, and clothing, the deceased would not be lacking those items in their next life. The bodies of the Chinese were later exhumed by a Chinese mortician who came to America for the purpose of returning the bones to China. By the 1880s, most of the Chinese had left Jacksonville. Some returned home and others went to work on the railroads. Those who stayed worked in private homes, laundries, or restaurants.

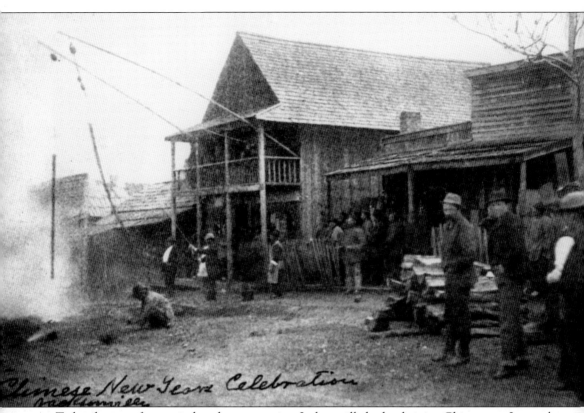

Chinese New Year Celebration
Jacksonville

Today there are few reminders that at one time Jacksonville had a thriving Chinatown. Located on Main Street, Chinatown consisted of wooden shacks as pictured above. The Chinese arrived in America in search of the same thing that had brought men from all over the world to the small town of Jacksonville—GOLD! However, many of the white settlers discriminated against the Chinese. They were not allowed to own property, they were taxed at much greater rates than the whites, and they could not purchase a mining claim until it had been abandoned by a white man. The Chinese pictured here are celebrating Chinese New Year with firecrackers and joss sticks.

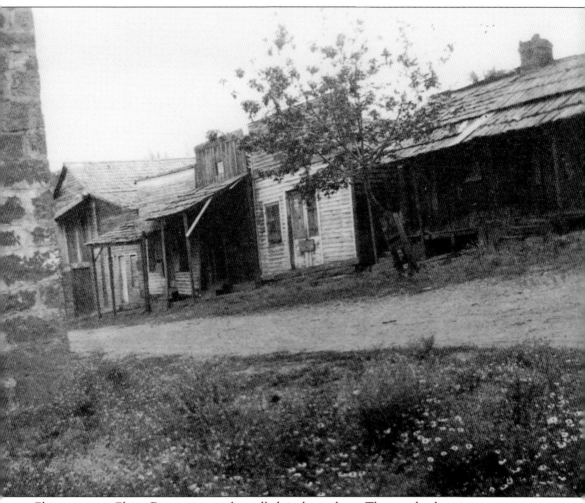

Chinatown, or China Row as it was also called, is shown here. The wooden housing structures served the basic purpose of keeping the elements out. The houses were propped up on whatever wood was available. The Chinese crowded into these small structures and were grateful for the opportunity to work in America in the hopes of making a better life for their families back home. They were a tight-knit group who could count on one another. They maintained their Chinese customs and ignored those who were vocal in opposition to their lifestyle.

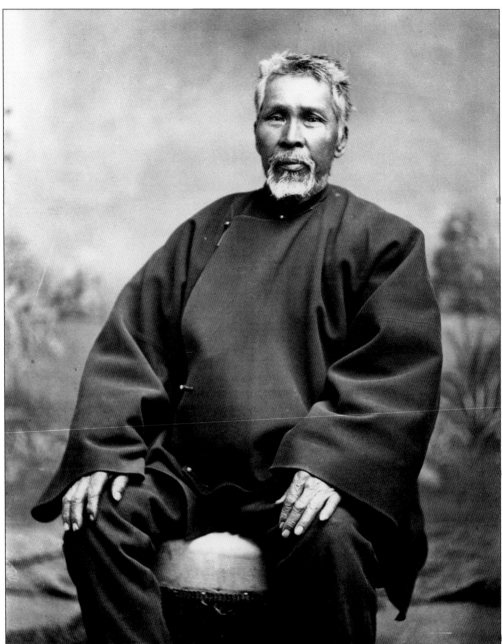

The Chinese men who came to America were employed by a Chinese boss. Pictured here is one such boss, Gin Lin. Lin contracted with white settlers who had large mining operations to provide them with laborers. Lin paid his laborers money but deducted what they owed him for their passage to America and their food and shelter once in America. Lin became very wealthy and was able to purchase his own mining claims regardless of the laws that prohibited Chinese from purchasing mining claims. In 1864, Lin paid $900 for land near the Little Applegate River and Sterling Creek. He purchased other parcels of land, amassing more wealth. Lin is credited with introducing hydraulic mining to the Applegate valley just outside of Jacksonville. Today the Gin Lin hiking trail takes visitors past some of the areas the Chinese mined so long ago.

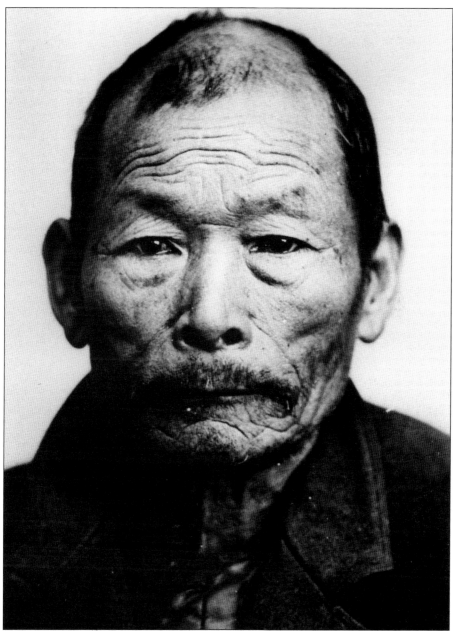

The photograph above is of Lin Wang. He operated a Chinese laundry on California Street between Third and Fourth Streets. Chinese businessmen were taxed at a rate of $50 per month beginning in the 1850s. Chinese miners were taxed $2 per month. The local newspaper, the *Oregon Sentinel*, ran a story on September 1, 1866, saying, "It seems an unwise policy to allow a race of brutish heathen who have nothing in common with us, to exhaust our mineral lands without paying a heavy tax for their occupation." In the 1880s, Jacksonville passed an ordinance that read: Every person or persons who shall set up or keep as a business, any washhouse or laundry within the corporate limits of Jacksonville shall pay a quarterly license of no less than five dollars for keeping or setting up such a business. No other service business in Jacksonville was taxed in a similar manner.

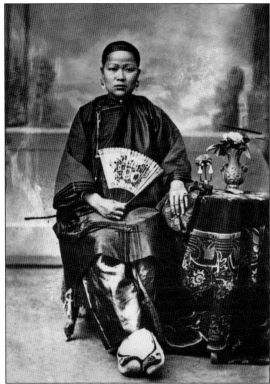

There were not many Chinese women in Jacksonville. Most of the females stayed behind in China to raise the children while the men made the journey to America. These women were photographed by Peter Britt in his studio. All Chinese women in Jacksonville wore trousers similar to those worn by Chinese men. The trousers were usually blue in color and made of cotton cloth. The women adorned their hair with a silver pin or a flower. They did not wear hats as the white women did but instead placed either a band of velvet or a small handkerchief around their heads.

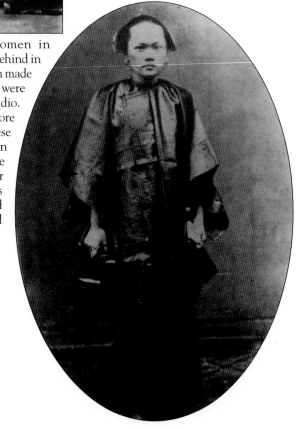

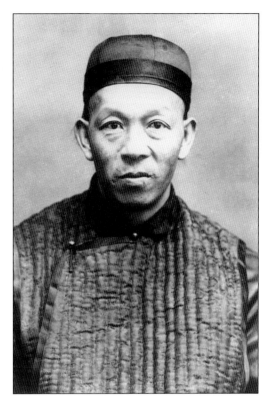

It was common for the Chinese men to wear skullcaps as pictured at right. Their clothing generally consisted of blue pants, a long jacket, white stockings, and lightweight shoes. Many of the men kept their hair short in the front and long in the back, known as a "queue." Some of the white settlers ridiculed the appearance of the Chinese men who remained true to their native dress.

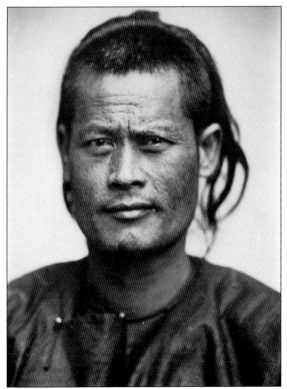

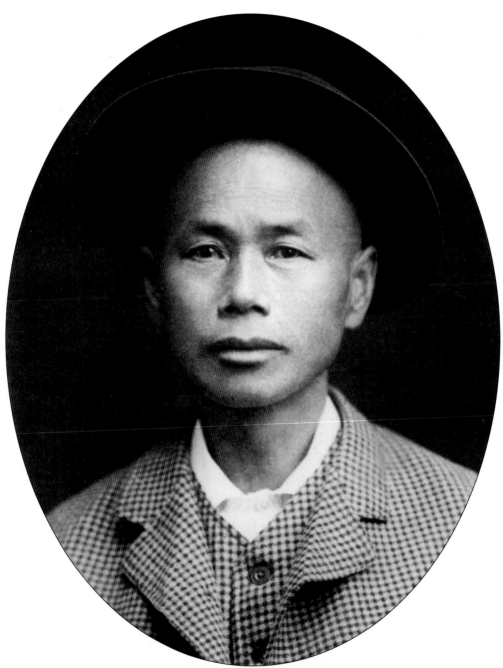

The gentleman pictured above is Yan, who worked for many years as a cook for the Beekman family. He was quite attached to the Beekmans and told the neighbors that when the Beekmans were away he missed them and was lonesome. The Southern Oregon Historical Society maintains a large collection of correspondence from the family and one letter states, "Yan was delighted to see us, had a bright fire in the sitting room, and a nice supper prepared for us which we ate with keen relish." Another letter refers to the family returning after travelling and says, "Yan, faithful boy, took good care of my birds and flowers for me. He says the time was very long to him and he was very lonesome."

Peter Britt was friendly to the Chinese during the time that many whites discriminated against them. Britt hired many Chinese to work in his gardens and his home. He loaned them money so they could start businesses. Above all, he treated them with respect. Britt took numerous photographs of the Chinese as evidenced here. Although these individuals are not identified, we can appreciate their clothing and accessories.

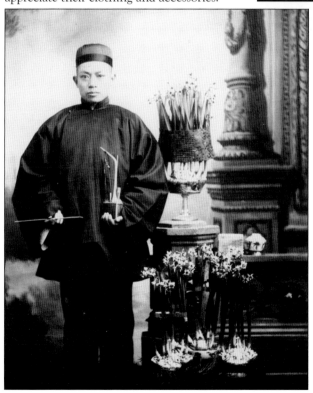

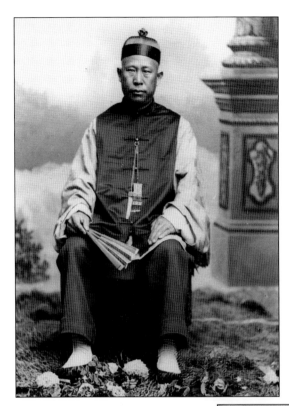

The Chinese man pictured at left is in traditional dress. He is having his portrait taken by Peter Britt. Below is a ledger from Kasper Kubli's store outside of Jacksonville showing items purchased by Wanng Tonn, a miner. The merchandise sold included oil for 75¢, nails for 25¢, a shovel for $1.62, salt for 50¢, beans for 25¢, sugar for 25¢, whiskey for 62¢, tobacco for 50¢, butter for $1, garlic for 25¢, matches for 75¢, 1 pair of boots for $5.75, 2 pairs of pants for $4, 1 shirt for $1, and a hat for $3.75.

MARRIAGE CERTIFICATE.

STATE OF OREGON, } ss.
COUNTY OF JACKSON.

This is to certify that the undersigned *E. B. Watson* .... by authority of a License bearing date the *2d* day of *May* A. D. 18*73*, and issued by the County Clerk of the County of Jackson, did, on the *2d* day of *May* A. D. 18*73*, at the ~~house of~~ *Clerks office at Jacksonville* in the County and State aforesaid, join in Lawful Wedlock *Hung* of the County ~~of~~ of *Jackson*, and State of *Oregon*, and *Eu Yoi* of the County of *Jackson* and State of *Oregon*, with their mutual assent, in presence of *C. C. Beekman* and *L. L. McKenzie*, witnesses.

Witness my hand

E. B. Watson
County Judge

This marriage certificate dated May 2, 1873, joins a Chinese man by the name of Hung to a Chinese woman by the name of Eu Yoi. There were not very many Chinese women in Jacksonville, as most of the Chinese men had made the journey alone.

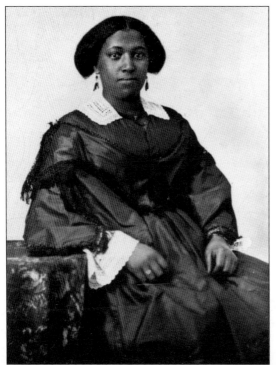

The names of those pictured here are unknown, but we do know there was a small population of African Americans living in Jacksonville or the nearby Kanaka Flats during the early days. Some black men came to Oregon alone hoping for a chance at freedom and others came enslaved with their owners. The Oregon Territory government excluded African Americans, and things were not any better when Oregon became a state in 1859. The state constitution stated that no African Americans could reside or be within the state, hold any real estate, make any contracts, or maintain any suit. The constitution also stipulated that no persons could bring African Americans into the state, employ them, or harbor them. The photograph of the young woman at left was taken in Peter Britt's studio.

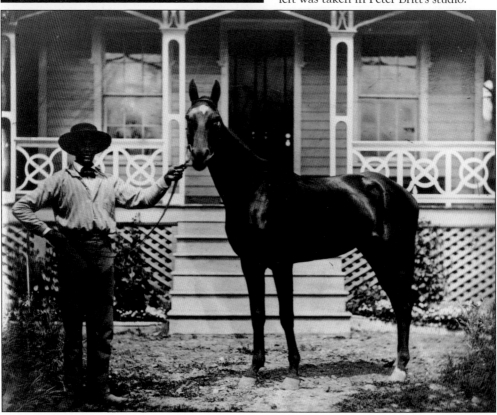

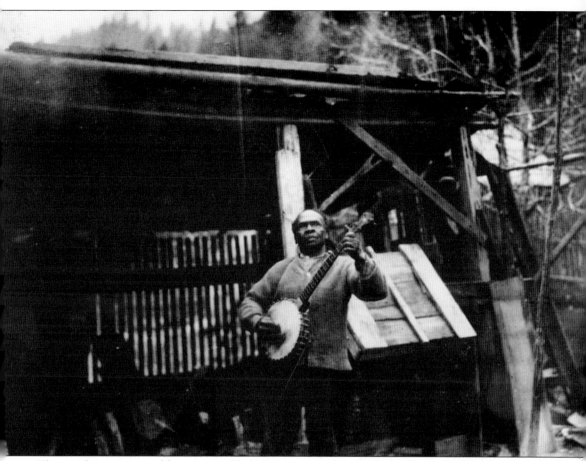

The gentleman pictured here is possibly living just outside of Jacksonville in the Kanaka Flats. The house he is standing in front of is just basic shelter to keep out the elements. Kanaka Flats was home to many "men of color," as they were called at the time, which included African Americans, Hispanics, and Hawaiians.

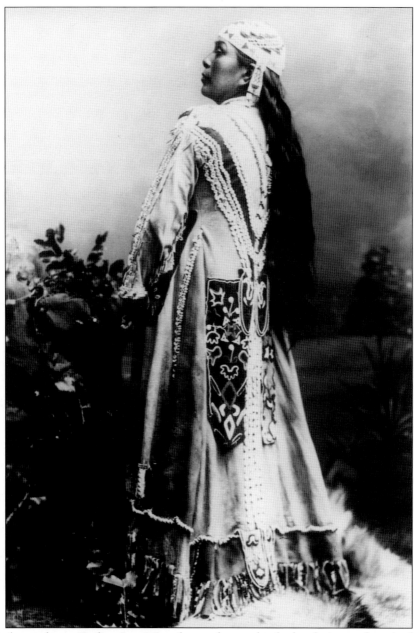

Lady Oscharwasha, or "Indian Jennie" as she was known by the locals, is seen here in the burial robe that she labored over for months prior to her death. Sensing her time was near and being the last survivor of her tribe, the Takelma Indians, she began to make her own burial robe. It was made from buckskin and adorned with colorful beads, seashells, transparent pebbles, small coins, and other ornaments. By the time she was finished, the robe weighed an estimated 50 pounds. She was offered money for the robe and was even offered money to show it at the Chicago World's Fair, but she refused all offers. When she died on May 14, 1893, a local newspaper, the *Democratic Times*, reported, "There was something extremely pathetic in the sole survivor thus respecting the traditions of her tribe in making such elaborate preparations for her interment as the last of the royal line. Let her remains rest in peace."

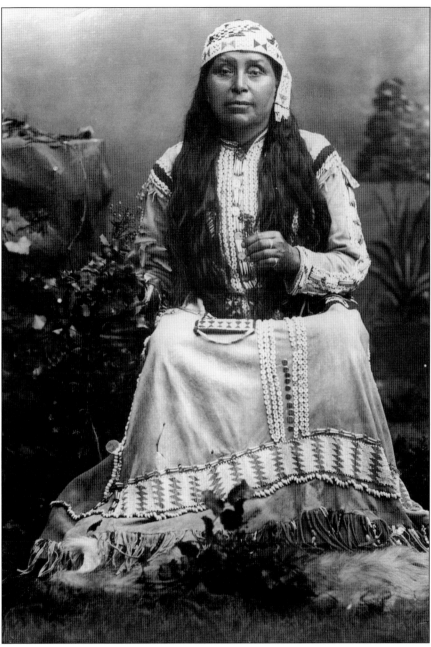

Indian Jennie is pictured here in her burial robe in Peter Britt's studio. As a young woman during the Rogue Indian Wars, Jennie and approximately a dozen other Native American women were instrumental in keeping the peace. The women were liaisons between the white soldiers at Fort Lane and the Native Americans. They tried to convince the Native Americans that even if they were triumphant, it would be short lived because the white settlers would continue to come in to the valley and the Native Americans would be outnumbered. Gen. Lindsay Applegate credited the women for paving the way for the first peace treaty signed in 1853. Indian Jennie was one of the few members of her tribe who remained in the valley after the local Native Americans were led to the Siletz Reservation. Indian Jennie lived out her days in Jacksonville.

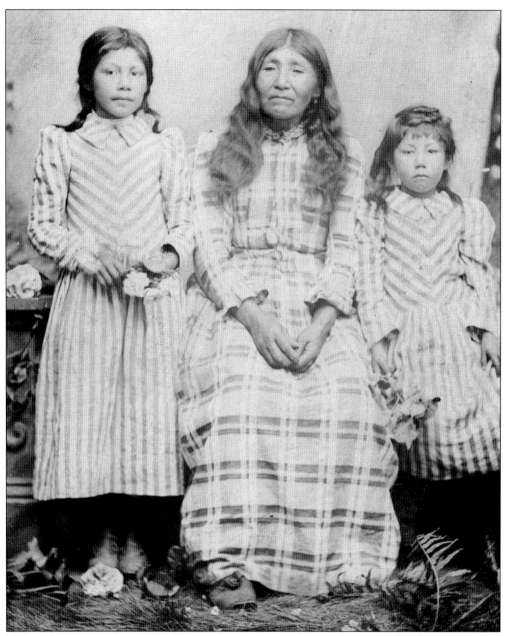

She was known simply as Indian Mary. Mary is pictured here with her two daughters. Mary was one of a handful of women who stayed behind when the Native Americans were marched off to the Siletz Reservation in 1856. On September 6, 1884, a local newspaper, the *Oregon Sentinel*, reported, "Old Mary, an Indian woman who has been living here since the first settlement of the country is seriously sick and no longer able to maintain herself. She has for the last thirty years been washing and doing light work around Jacksonville and has always earned her living and now that she is no longer able to work she should be properly cared for in her old age and sickness. The Indians have all gone from here and there is no one to care for the poor old destitute woman unless our people do something for her and as she has succeeded in taking care of herself through all these years, we think she deserves some consideration at our hands."

Three

THE LATER YEARS

In 1883, the railroad bypassed Jacksonville in favor of the newly formed town of Middleford, later renamed Medford. Jacksonville residents did not appreciate this and began referring to their rival as Mudville, Rabbit Hole, and the like. Jacksonville had been the hub of all activity and did not take kindly to playing second fiddle to Medford. Some business owners packed up and moved to Medford and many residents followed suit. Jacksonville became a sleepy little town while Medford introduced theatres with live entertainment and then talkie movies, a Carnegie Library, and many stores. The death knell sounded for Jacksonville when the voters decided to move the county seat to Medford in 1927. The ensuing years brought the Great Depression, World War II, the Korean War, and the Vietnam War, which just pushed Jacksonville further into oblivion. There were few job opportunities for the locals. In the mid- to late-1960s, plans were made to bulldoze the downtown core in favor of a new highway. The locals took a good look around and realized they had something unique that could not be replaced. In 1967, the U.S. Hotel was restored and that sparked an interest in the town that time forgot. Within a short time, more than 100 buildings were restored and placed on the National Historic Registry. Today the entire town of Jacksonville is a Historic Landmark District.

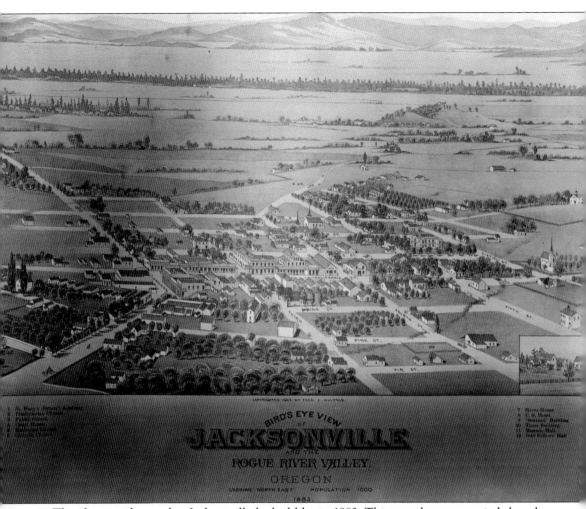

This drawing shows what Jacksonville looked like in 1883. This was the same period that the railroad bypassed Jacksonville in favor of the land shown out in the distance. That land soon became the town of Middleford, later renamed Medford. Those in Jacksonville preferred to call it Mudville and Rabbit Hole. The Jacksonville school can be seen in the far right corner, and just below that is the Presbyterian Church. Although there were still some Chinese living in Jacksonville at the time, not much was left of Chinatown by 1883. The downtown core is much as it appears today with the U.S. Hotel, the Masonic building, the Odd Fellows building, and the Orth building.

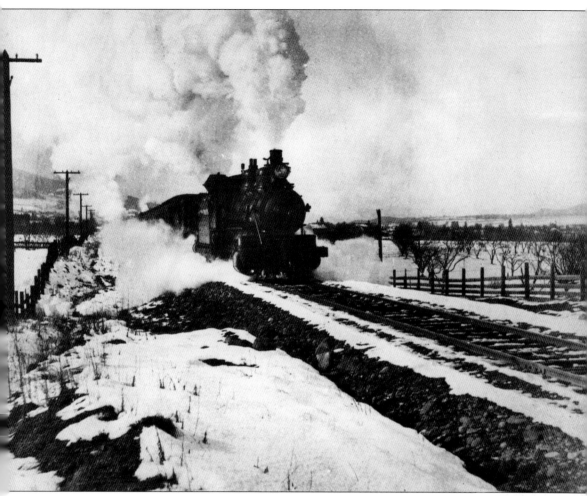

The coming of the railroad was great news for most towns. It meant job opportunities and a new way to travel. The lush interiors of a train car were a far cry from the bumpy, dusty rides of a stagecoach. You were no longer at the mercy of a team of horses, but instead you could ride in luxury and at a much faster pace. However, the advent of the railroad meant the end of an era for the small community of Jacksonville. Jacksonville had always been the main hub, but when the railroad passed it by and instead chose the nearby town of Middleford, it sounded the death knell for the bustling town of Jacksonville. The railroad line began in Portland and came as far south as Roseburg. It needed to get down to Ashland to accommodate two mills there. There was no room in Jacksonville for a turnaround, so the railroad authorities decided Middleford was the better option. With that, Middleford became the bustling city and Jacksonville began playing second fiddle.

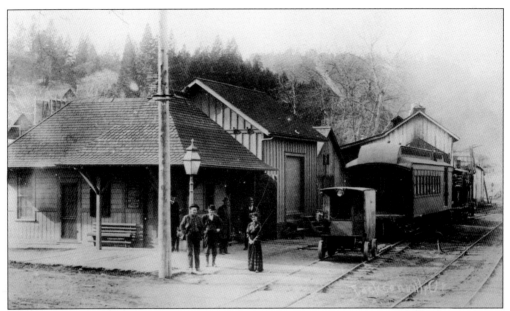

Immediately after losing the railroad to Medford, the citizens of Jacksonville saw the need for a railroad spur that would connect the two towns. Despite the need for a small train, it was years before it became a reality. The Rogue River Valley Railway Company was formed, but financial success eluded the company. Difficulties abounded, including the ability to stay on track, and the train was dubbed the "Jacksonville Cannonball." In 1893, the business was leased to William Barnum. The photo above shows the small train alongside the depot in Jacksonville, and the photo below shows William Barnum and his oldest son, John, inside the depot. The Rogue River Valley Railway Company was not known for its reliability; therefore, many of the townsfolk joked that it was operated by the Father, the Son, and the Holy Ghost.

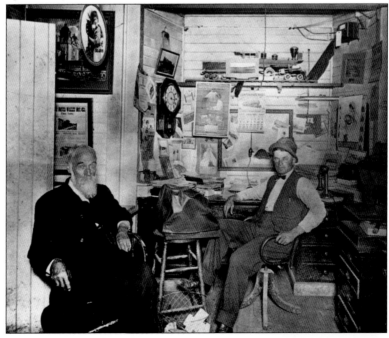

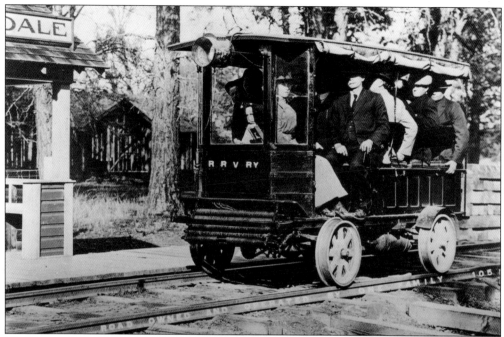

The Rogue River Valley Railway Company added an "auto car" to the line that ran between Jacksonville and Medford at a cost of 25¢ for the 15-minute ride to Medford. The photograph above shows the car crowded with passengers. The Rogue River Valley Railway Company continued to struggle through the years, and the 20th century brought such things as automobiles into the picture. In 1915, the Southern Oregon Traction Company purchased the company. They electrified the line and operated an electric car between the towns. By the early 1920s, it was obvious that the "little engine that could" was never going to be successful. In 1928, the tracks between the two towns were removed.

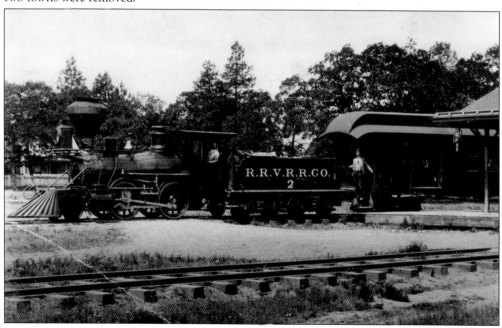

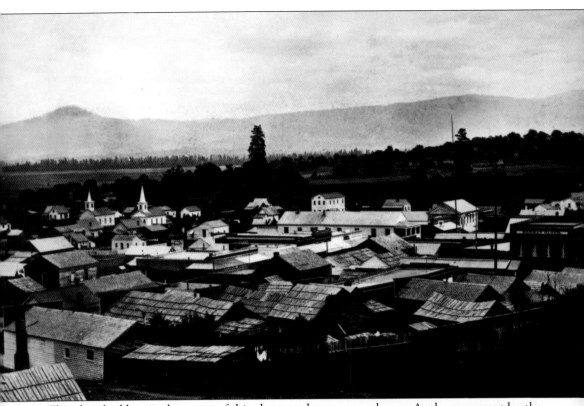

The white building in the center of this photograph was a courthouse. As the years went by, the townsfolk wanted to replace the white building. By 1869, the local newspaper posed the question, "Is Jackson County so poor it cannot afford a decent courthouse?" Ten years went by and another local newspaper stated, "This dilapidated old structure is a disgrace to the county." Another ten years passed and the local newspaper stated, "Is it not time that the county had a courthouse that would not be mistaken by a stranger for a barn?" A grand jury report dated December 1881 stated, "There are stables and barns in this state more creditable in appearance than the Courthouse of Jackson County, and our county court should build one as a matter of public duty." The following year, the county commissioners voted two to one to build a new courthouse. In 1883, construction began on the two-story brick building that still stands today.

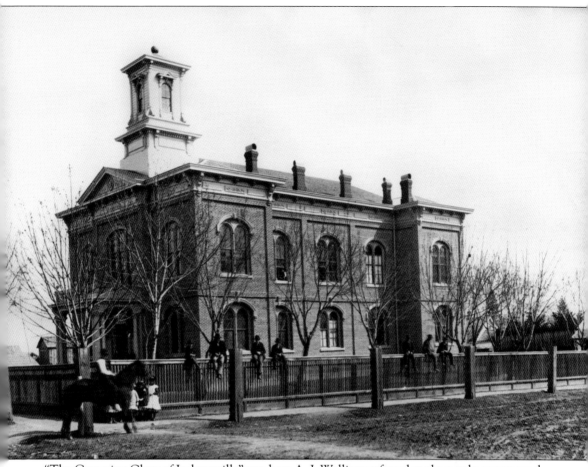

"The Crowning Glory of Jacksonville" was how A. J. Wallings referred to the newly constructed Jacksonville Courthouse in 1883. That expression still holds true today. The cost to construct the building was $32,000. The building was not even finished when the local residents decided to throw a grand ball on New Year's Eve. Horse and buggies lined the street, bringing the townsfolk who were dressed in their finest clothing to a ball at the construction site of their new courthouse. In 1927, the county seat moved to Medford and the courthouse stood still and empty. One local resident, Helen Colvig Cook, reminisced about what the courthouse had meant to her by saying, "Many of us who knew it when it was young and proud and we were young too, knew it was not only as a courthouse, in one sense of the word, but in another sense as well. For having no other park, in the town, its large yard shaded by splendid maples, served as a meeting place and trysting place for the young people of the community."

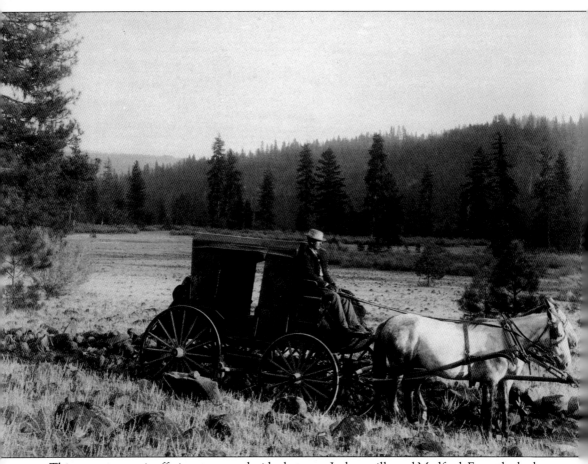
This entrepreneur is offering stagecoach rides between Jacksonville and Medford. From the looks of this set up it appears that it would have been a long and difficult journey compared to today.

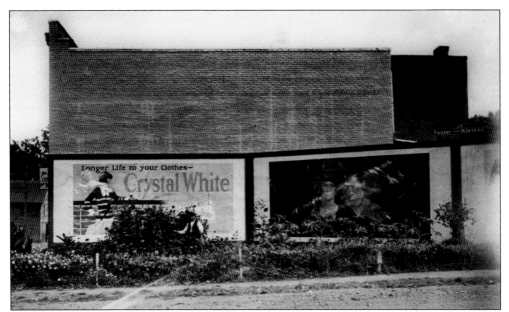

By the late 1800s, wall graphics began appearing on buildings in Jacksonville and around the country. If a building was not available, then a barn would do. The wall graphics were used to advertise a product or to promote a business. Hotels would use them to list not only their prices but also any special features such as a bath. It was not uncommon to see wall graphics promoting a certain beer or whiskey on the side of the local watering hole. The people who painted the graphics were called "wall dogs," and they would travel around the country painting the advertisements. Wall graphics fell out of favor in the 1920s as the country purchased automobiles and advertisements began to appear along the roads. Today in Jacksonville, you can still see graphics that date to the late 1800s.

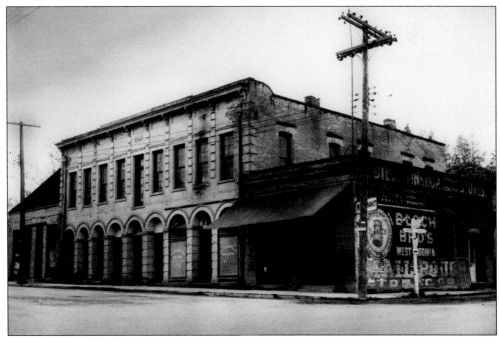

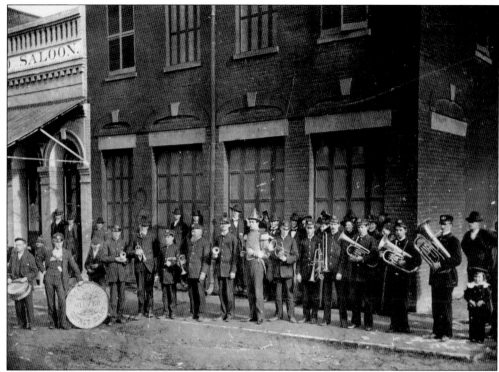

The Jacksonville Silver Cornet Band was in demand in the 1880s. They played at weddings, reunions, and community events. In 1885, the band's director, Herr Schmid, told a local newspaper, the *Oregon Sentinel*, he had sent away for some new music and "The champion band of Oregon" would soon have some new numbers to entertain the crowds. When the Helman Red Suit Band from Ashland got new uniforms, the Jacksonville Silver Cornet Band decided they needed new uniforms in order to stay competitive. A masquerade ball was held on February 14, 1885, at the U.S. Hotel ballroom. It was well attended and brought in a good sum of money. The band held a few more fundraisers and was able to purchase new uniforms as well as a wagon.

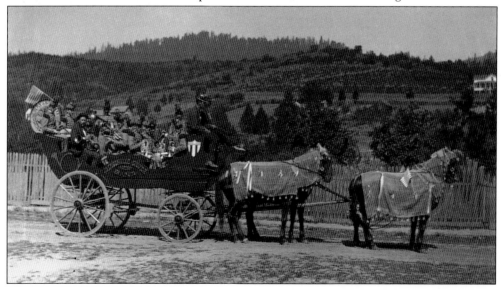

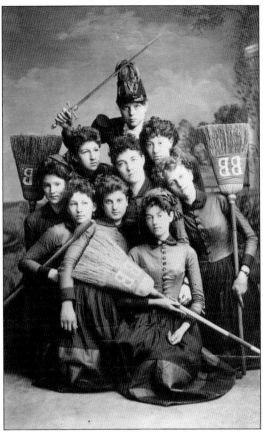

During the late 1800s, Broom Brigades became popular activities for young girls across America. It was thought to be an activity in which girls could excel and which would teach them drills similar to what males were learning in the military. These photographs of the Jacksonville Broom Brigade were taken in 1888. The girls were expected to be able to maneuver their brooms in poses similar to what men did with their guns. The girls practiced many poses, from standing straight to kneeling with the broom. The Jacksonville Broom Brigade wore costumes and spent many hours practicing.

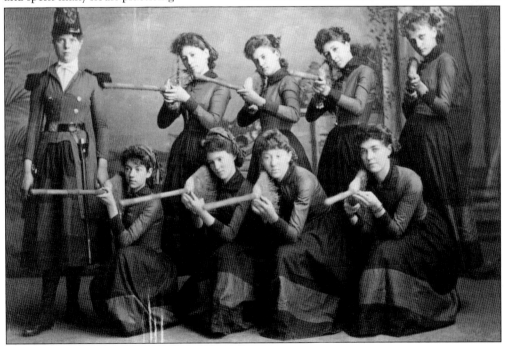

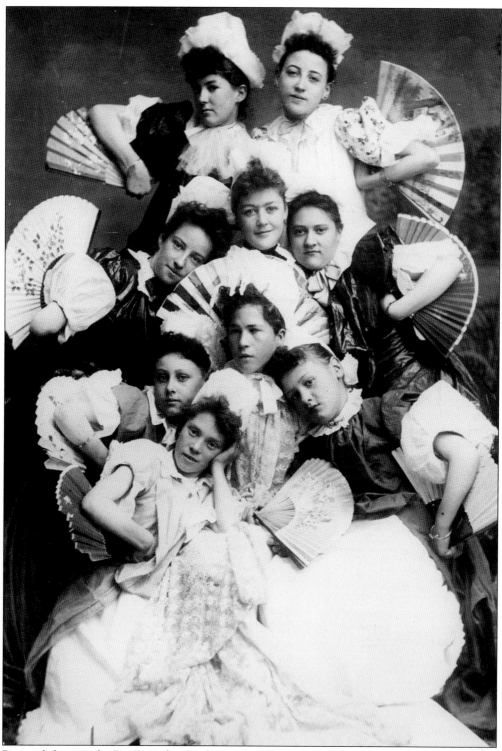

Pictured above is the Fan Brigade of Jacksonville. These young ladies practiced maneuvers with their fans similar to what the girls who participated in Jacksonville's Broom Brigade learned.

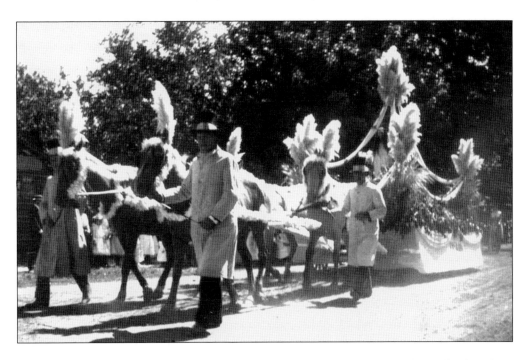

It has been said that everyone loves a parade, and apparently that was true in Jacksonville when these photographs were taken in 1895. The Native Sons of Oregon created the float pictured below.

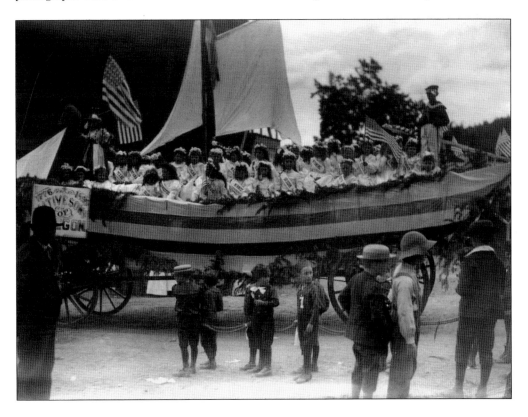

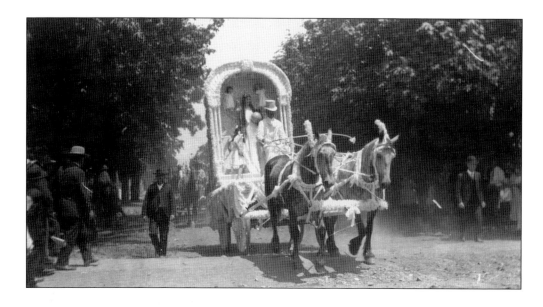

The residents of Jacksonville took their parades quite seriously, as evidenced here. The preparations that went into these floats are quite remarkable especially when we realize how busy the townsfolk were in their daily lives.

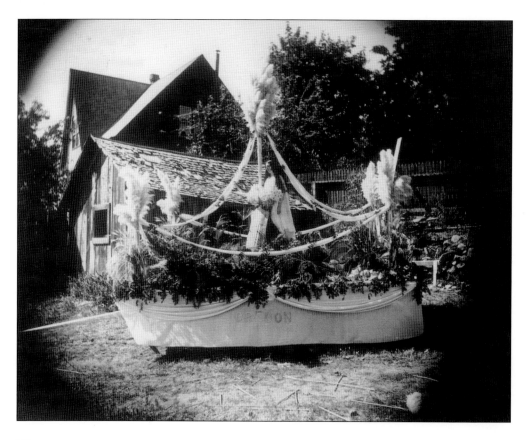

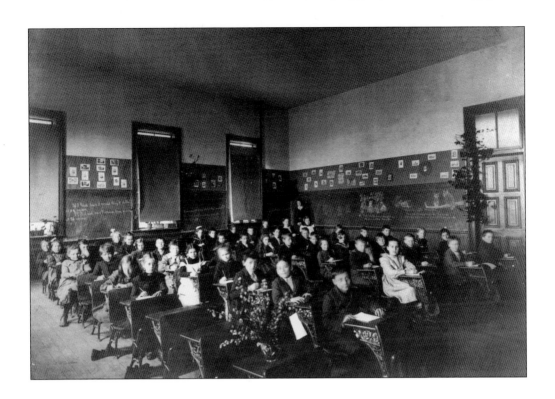

The students pictured here are hard at work. The picture below, taken in 1904, includes the teacher, Ms. Starry. Teachers in Jacksonville, as well as in other communities in America, were expected to be unmarried and above reproach. They were not to partake of alcohol or gambling. It was common for the town's schoolteacher to board with a family.

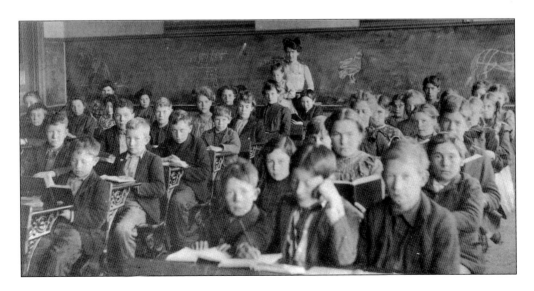

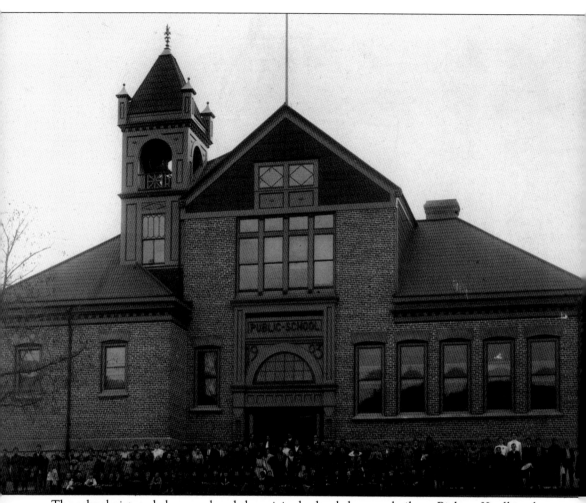
The school pictured above replaced the original school that was built on Bigham Knoll in the 1860s. That school burned to the ground on January 25, 1903. The cause of the fire was never determined. While this new school was being built, classes were held in churches, assembly halls, and the local brewery.

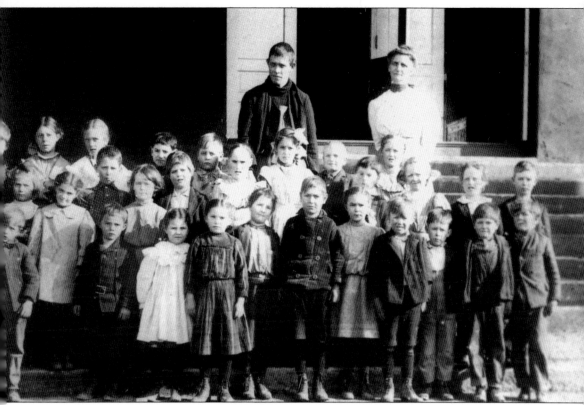

The first and second grade class of 1908–1909 is pictured here with their teacher and principal. At that time, there was one playground for the boys and another for the girls. George Wendt remembered playing such games as bullfrog, skating in the mud, marbles, spinning tops, football, baseball, or "just standing around eating apples." Games for the girls included jumping rope, hopscotch, tag, and drop the handkerchief.

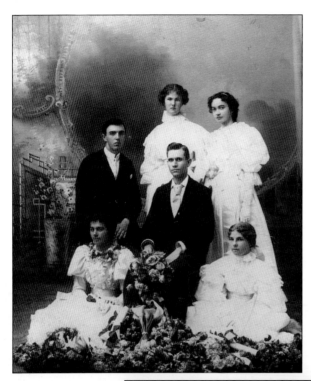

Graduation from eighth grade was taken very seriously, as these photographs show. For some students, graduating from the eighth grade was the end of their scholastic career, but others would go on to receive additional schooling. The Jacksonville School was kindergarten through the eighth grade when these young people were students there.

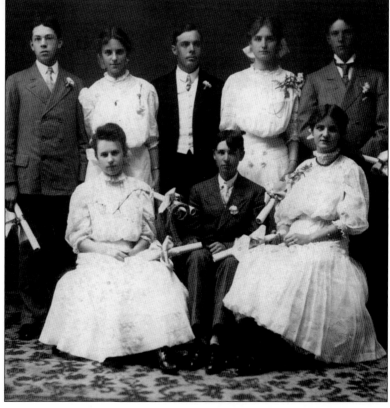

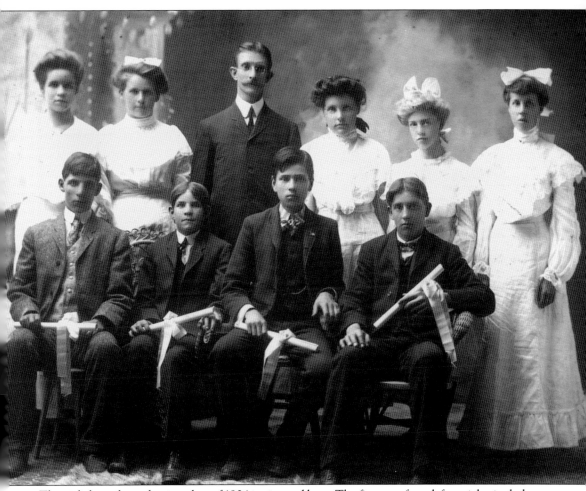

The eighth grade graduating class of 1904 is pictured here. The first row, from left to right, includes Earl Peter, Holman Peter, Richard Gaskins, and Almond S. Wilcox; the second row includes Mary Peter, Ida Fink, E. E. Washborn, Mabel Pruitt, Emma Wendt, and Abbie Henry.

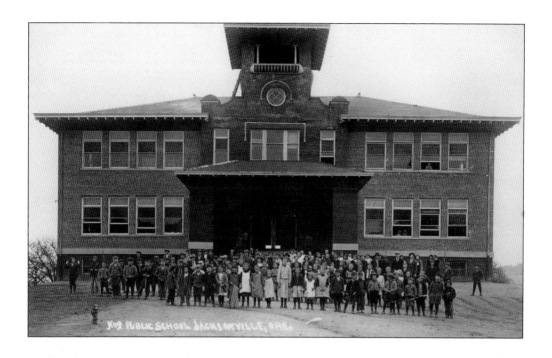

The school pictured here replaced the "fireproof school" built in 1903. That school burned on December 14, 1906, probably from a defective heater. This new school cost $20,000 and had electric lights and steam heating. A janitor chopped wood and supplied the system with enough water (about six gallons a day) to heat the two-story structure. The photograph below is from 1917.

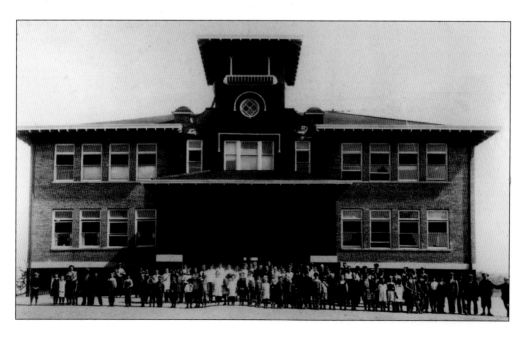

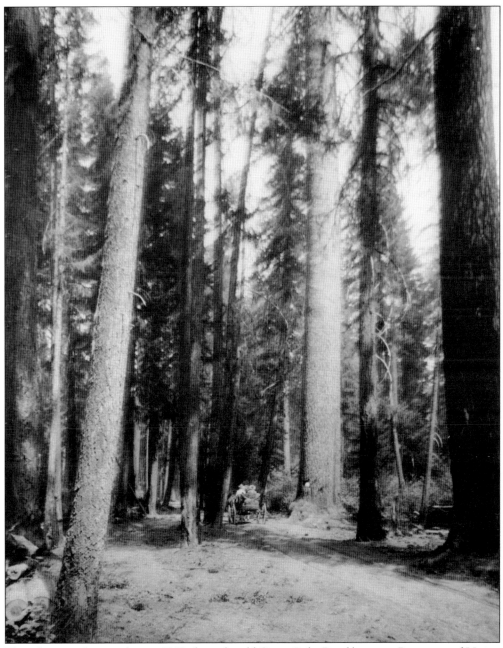
This photograph was taken in 1909 along the old Crater Lake Road between Prospect and Union Creek. Possibly the family was heading out to do some camping and enjoy the pristine scenery.

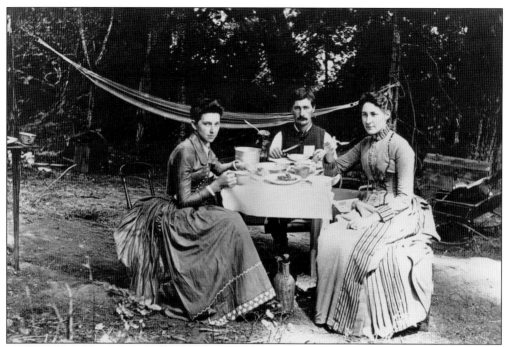

These campers seem to be enjoying their freshly made meal in a beautiful mountain setting. Camping took a great deal of planning, and the journey, although beautiful, could take a long time by horse and buggy. The campers pictured below seem to be enjoying their trip. Note the one female is holding a rifle as though she is ready to go out in search of that evening's meal.

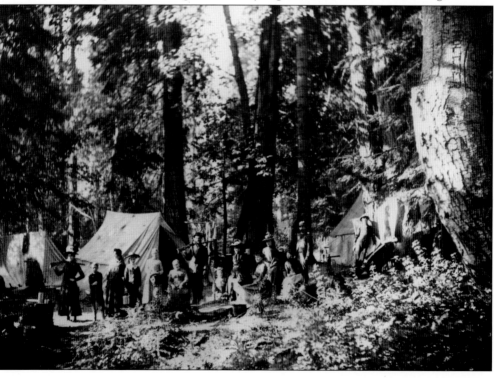

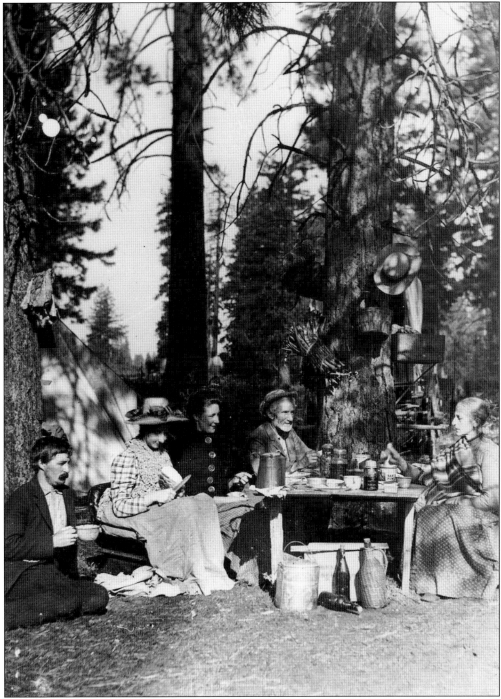

Emil Britt, pictured at the left with a coffee cup, and Mollie Britt, third from the left, are enjoying some time in the mountains with friends. Note their ingenious use of the tree as a hat rack of sorts.

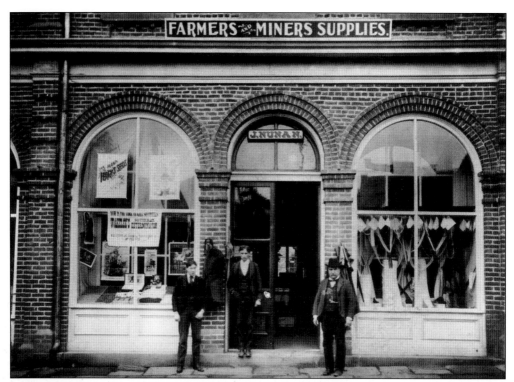

Jeremiah Nunan of Nunan, Taylor, and Company offered the community a bit of everything in his mercantile. He sold clothing for men and boys, fancy and dress goods, California made boots and shoes, hosiery and ribbons, men's and boy's straw hats, stationery, blank books, cigars and tobacco, crockery and glassware, and groceries and canned goods. A sampling of prices from 1904 include: a pound of butter for 55¢, 5 dozen eggs for $1, a pound of bacon for 40¢, a 17-pound ham for $2.90, 10 pounds of sugar for $6.45, 3 pounds of coffee for 90¢, and 50 pounds of potatoes for 75¢. Jeremiah also offered 20 pounds of nails for $1, 10 yards of gingham for $1, and 12 yards of calico for $75¢.

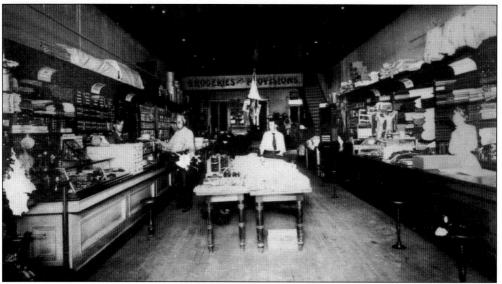

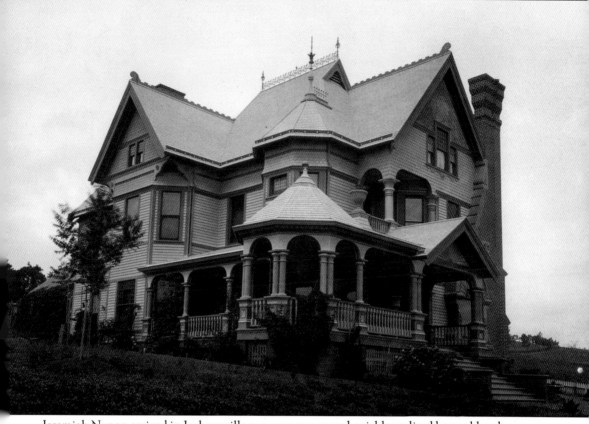

Jeremiah Nunan arrived in Jacksonville as a young man and quickly realized he could make more money operating a saddle and harness store than he could as a gold miner. He became friends with Henry Judge, who was in the same line of work. Henry had recently married Anna O'Grady, who had immigrated with her family to America from Ireland. Through that friendship, Jeremiah met Anna's sister, Delia. They began courting and were married on June 3, 1872, at St. Joseph's Catholic Church. Over the years, they had five children. In 1892 Jeremiah sent away for house plans from the George F. Barber catalog. In April of that year, construction began on what the local newspaper referred to as "The most elegant home in Jacksonville." The local newspaper frequently wrote about the various local contractors' progress on the home and who was furnishing the materials. The family moved into their new home in time for Christmas that year. Today, people in automobiles drive past the house admiring its beauty just as people in stagecoaches and buggies once did.

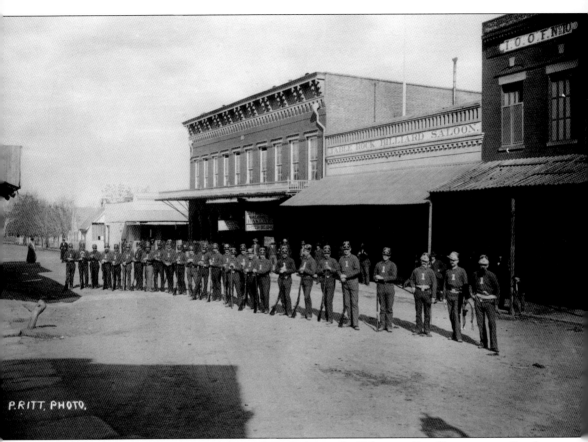

The photograph above shows 27 men of the Jacksonville Volunteer Fire Department. On the day this photograph was taken, they were charged with keeping the peace during the hanging of Lewis O'Neil. Lewis was accused of murdering Lewis McDaniel on November 20, 1884, in Ashland. McDaniel was shot to death on his way home after dark. Once his body was discovered, the townsfolk immediately began pointing towards O'Neil, citing his personal relationship with McDaniel's wife, Mandy. O'Neil denied the entire thing but was unable to provide an alibi. He admitted to owning a gun similar to the murder weapon but claimed he had sold his gun to a man in Gold Hill. O'Neil was not able to provide the authorities with the name of the man who had bought the weapon. It also did not help that O'Neil's shoe prints matched those in the snow at the scene of the crime. O'Neil was convicted of the murder and Judge Webster ordered that he be hanged on March 12, 1886.

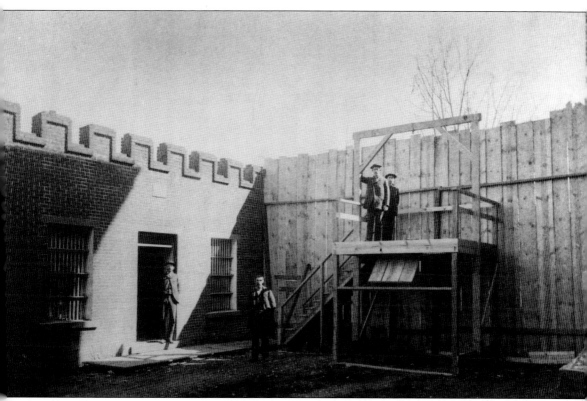

Judge Webster ordered that special gallows be built between the jail and the courthouse. The gallows were 40 by 60 feet with a 16-foot tight board fence surrounding it. The jail formed one wall of the fence, and the courthouse served as the other wall. As the crews worked building the gallows, O'Neil sat in his jail cell listening to each board being pounded into place.

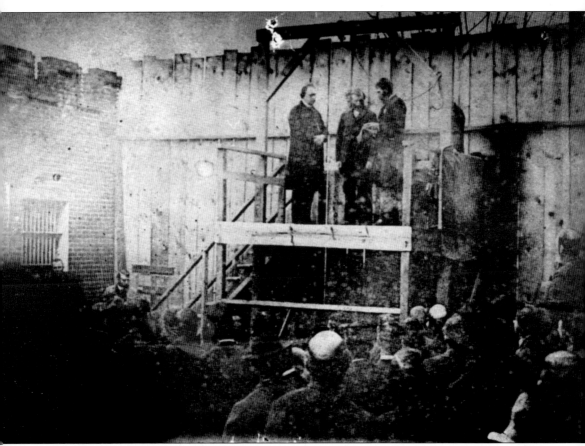

The day arrived and a crowd of approximately 200 people gathered to witness the event. Father Blanchet accompanied O'Neil to the gallows and when Sheriff Jacobs asked if O'Neil had any final words to say, it was Father Blanchet who replied that O'Neil did not. After the hanging, O'Neil was buried in the pauper section of the Jacksonville cemetery. The rope was cut into small pieces and distributed amongst the crowd.

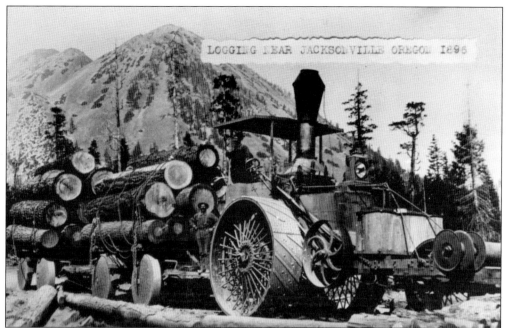

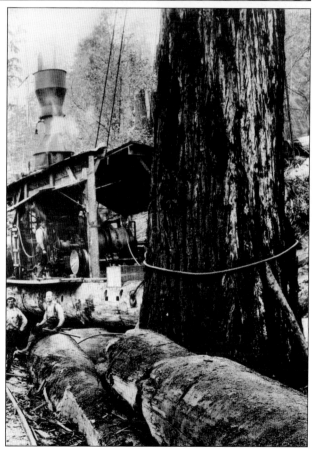

Logging began in earnest just outside of Jacksonville in the late 1800s and brought many job opportunities. The photograph above, taken in 1896, shows the tremendous equipment needed to haul the gigantic logs. The photograph at right shows the size of the logs the men were working with. Sawing and felling trees was dangerous work, as they did not have the safety equipment we have today.

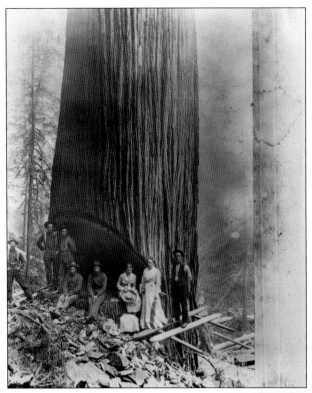

Many men living in Jacksonville worked in the logging industry in the late 1800s. Their work took them into southern Oregon and northern California where they swung their axes for days at a time trying to make some headway at felling trees the size of the ones in these photographs. The men would first chop just far enough into the tree so they could place a springboard about six feet off the ground all around the tree. Once the springboards were in place, they would stand on the springboards and chop away at the tree.

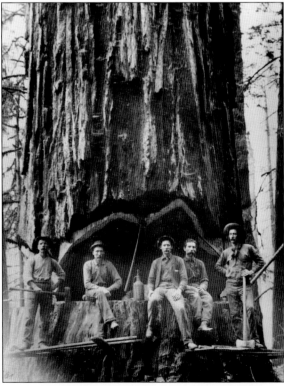

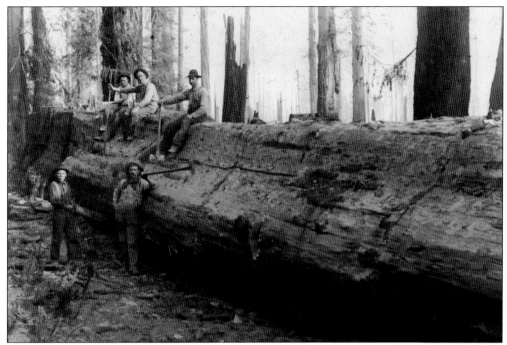

The men shown above have felled this tree and are now taking a much-needed break. They only had the most rudimentary tools for this massive job. It appears the women and children in the photograph below have come to offer their support to the man who is working to turn the logs into lumber to be used for building homes and other structures.

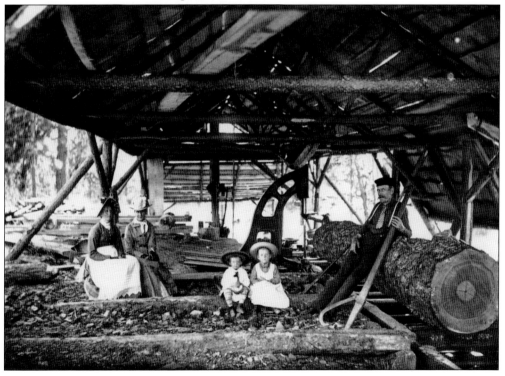

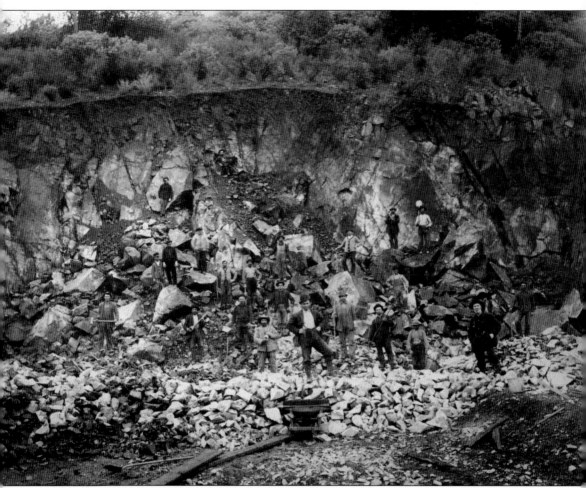

Many men in Jacksonville were employed at the Jacksonville Quarry in the early 1900s. The quarry was located one-fourth of a mile outside of Jacksonville. It was very dangerous work, and many men lost their lives or were badly injured while working there. They used black powder and dynamite to blast away at the hillside. When an injury or death occurred, a worker would use the telephone on site to summon help in Jacksonville, but response times were slow and the injured had to be taken all the way to the Sacred Heart Hospital in Medford.

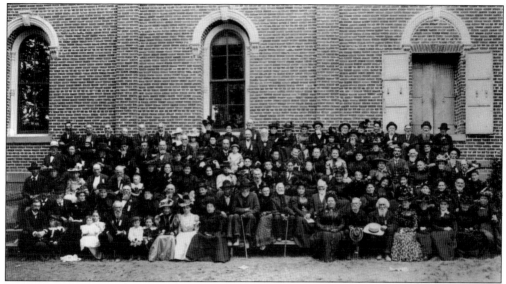

Once the pioneers reached Oregon and settled in, they realized the importance of what their journey would mean to future generations. They had come to Oregon seeking a better life for their families, and in doing so, they had made great sacrifices. What they had endured to reach Oregon, and what they did to settle the land upon arrival, would benefit generations of future Oregonians. Some of the pioneers decided to form a society known as the Pioneer Society, and soon the ranks grew until they had a large group as pictured here. They had meetings and social gatherings. They documented each member's personal history and wrote a nice story about each member upon their death. The Pioneer Society is pictured on the grounds of the Jacksonville Courthouse above; below they are enjoying a picnic.

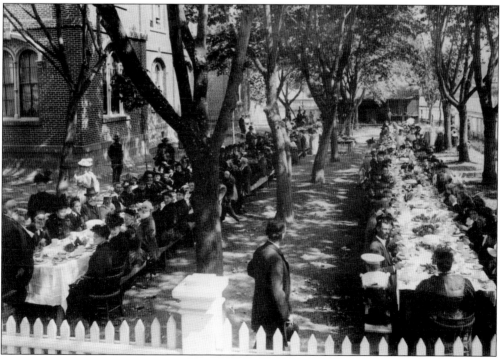

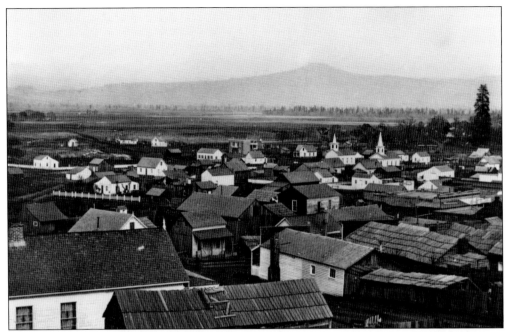

In the above early photograph of Jacksonville in the 1860s, there is nothing but pristine valley for as far as the eye can see. Roxy Ann Peak can be seen off in the distance. In the photograph below, taken in the early 1900s, the town of Medford is in the background directly under Roxy Ann Peak. A snow-capped Mount McLaughlin can be seen in the distance. The town of Jacksonville has spread out and the trees have grown and are now able to shade many of the homes.

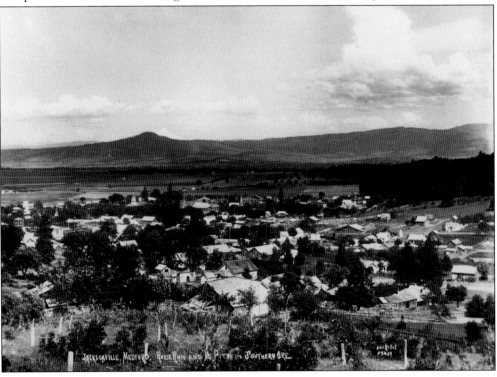

Ed Schieffelin was photographed by Peter Britt is his mining outfit. As a young boy, Ed grew up along the Rogue River but spent every minute he could panning for gold in Jacksonville and the surrounding area. Ed set his sights on a major strike, but that eluded him in this area. He moved to Arizona and it was there that he finally found his fortune. He struck a huge pocket of almost pure silver. Ed named the area Tombstone, and he and his brothers took out huge amounts of silver and gold from that area. He returned to the Rogue Valley still wanting to strike it rich here. Legend has it that he did find gold somewhere near Jacksonville but died before he could work the site. He is pictured below with his elaborate wagon pulled by his prized sorrels.

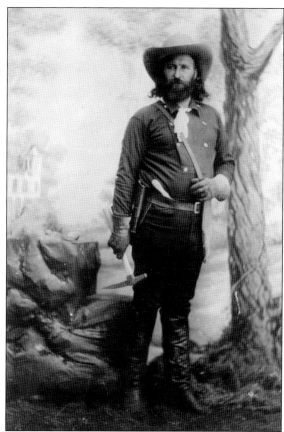

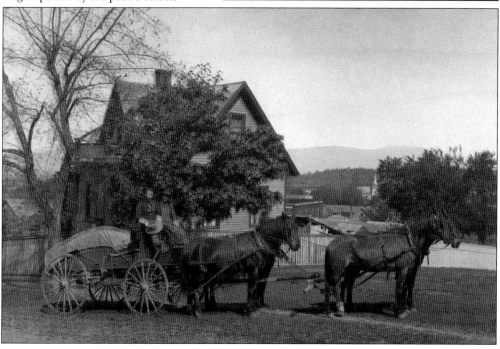

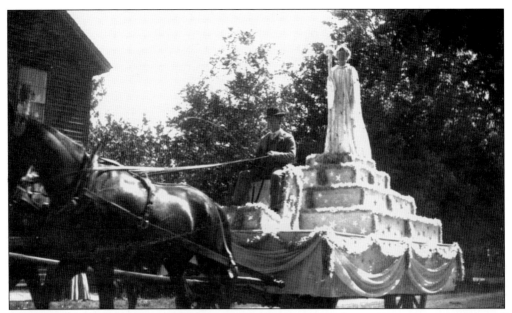

The Fourth of July parade in 1908 brought out the basic parade entries to the most fancy of parade entries. The young lady in white is on a float decorated as a large cake to celebrate the nation's birthday. The young girls with the wagon seem to be having a grand time entertaining the townsfolk along the parade route.

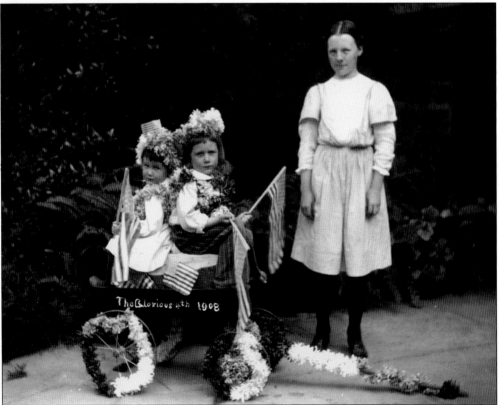

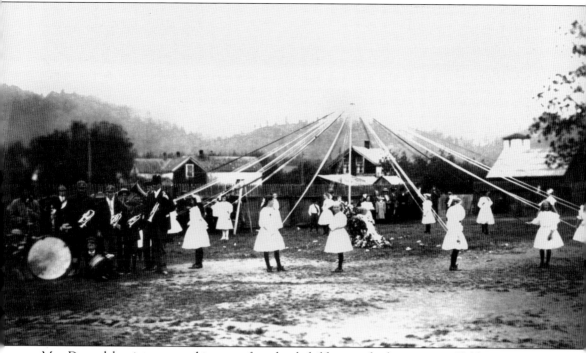

May Day celebrations were a big event for school children in the last century. Held every May 1st, the children danced around a maypole, as seen in this photograph taken around 1910 in Jacksonville. The band was playing in the background as the girls circled the maypole. Each year, one lucky girl was crowned "Queen of May." School children made baskets out of paper and placed flowers in the baskets. They would then leave the baskets of flowers on a neighbor's porch, ring the doorbell, and run away before someone had the chance to open the door.

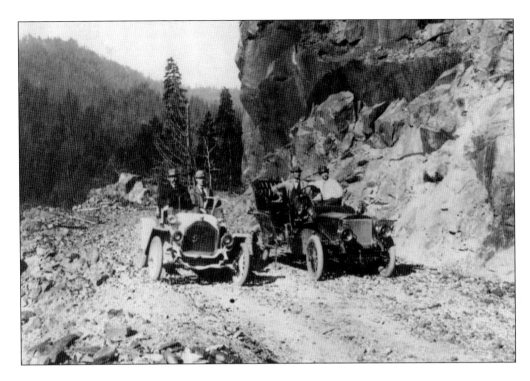

By 1910, a handful of people in Jacksonville owned automobile machines, as they were known at the time. The automobile brought many changes to towns across America, not least of which was the freedom to explore new places, as these people seem to be doing.

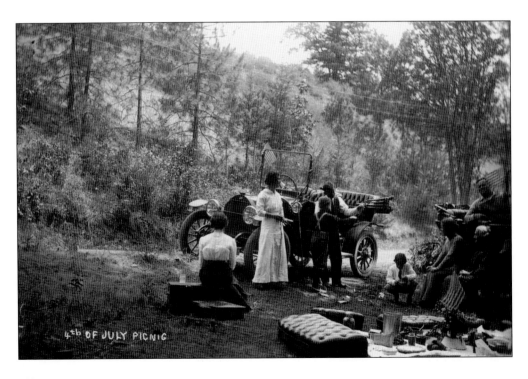

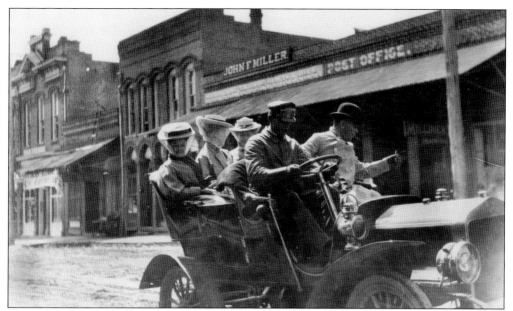

A ride in an automobile was an exciting adventure. However, the roads had not been paved yet so the automobiles had to drive through dirt and mud. Coats known as "dusters" were sold to men and women who wanted to keep the dust and dirt off their clothes.

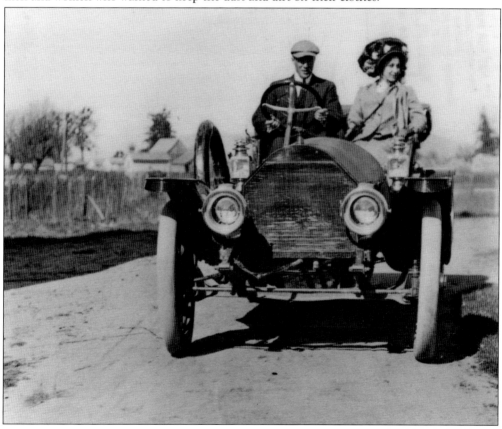

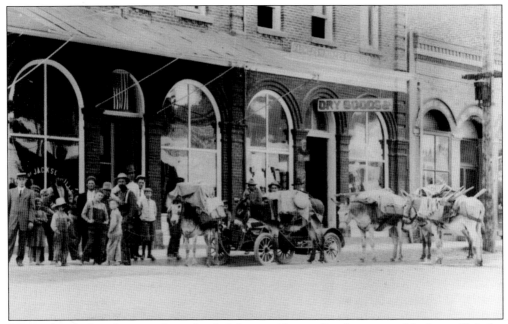

The mules in this photograph are loaded down with supplies from one of Jacksonville's dry goods stores. Just behind the mules is one of those newfangled automobile machines. The mules seem determined to show they will outlast this latest invention and will always be available to transport goods.

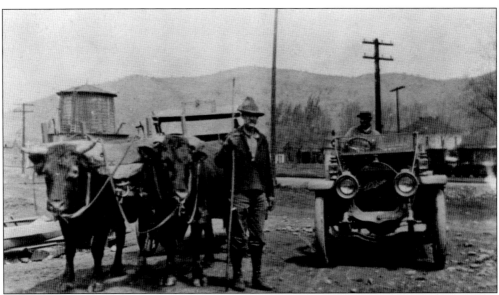

Perhaps in an effort to prove that newer does not always mean better, the gentleman on the left is walking beside his wagon pulled by oxen. The gentleman on the right seems rather amused at the sight as he sits perched in his new automobile machine.

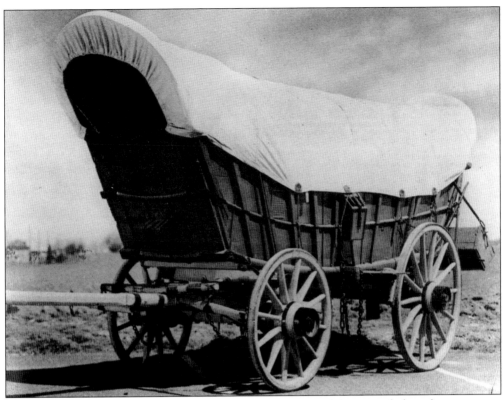

Many pioneers experienced tremendous changes during their lifetime including the inventions of electricity and indoor plumbing. Just in transportation alone, they saw the covered wagon, the horse and buggy, the stagecoach, the railroads, trolleys, and finally the automobile. Some even had the opportunity to see an actual flying machine, or what we refer to today as an airplane. On June 4, 1911, many Jacksonville residents took the train to Medford to watch as Eugene Ely took to the skies. He reached elevations of 600 to 2,000 feet. The crowd was thrilled to see such a sight, something that most could never have imagined.

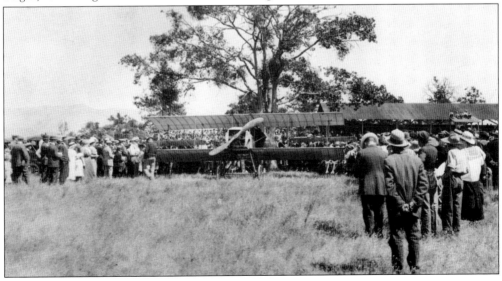

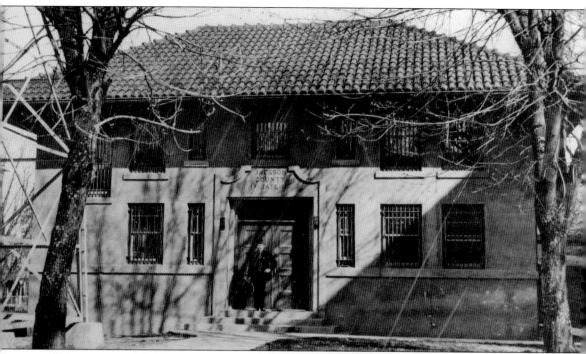

As long as there have been jails in Jacksonville, there have been prisoners with thoughts of a great escape. In 1875, a new jail was built to replace a simple rustic one. The local newspaper, the *Oregon Sentinel*, stated, "From the manner in which it is being built, it seems hardly possible for a person to get out, after once being locked up in one of those cells." Soon afterward, the *Oregon Sentinel* reported, "A new jail and two or three men guarding it, and yet a prisoner leaves in broad daylight." The jail pictured above was built in 1911 and was not without its share of escapes. In 1917, a prisoner, J. L. Ragsdale, hit Jailer Charles Bayse over the head with a flatiron. Ragsdale fled the jail taking another prisoner as a hostage. Three men and four young boys gave chase. Sheriff Jennings and 30 National Guardsmen quickly surrounded the area. Realizing there was no escape, Ragsdale used the gun he had stolen from Bayse and took his own life. Bayse died within hours of the attack.

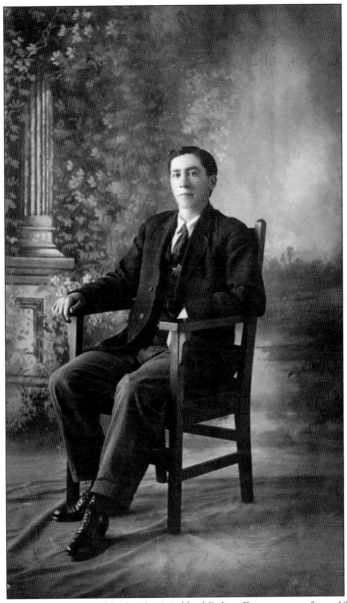

August Singler worked as a constable for the Medford Police Department from 1909 to 1913. He earned the nickname of "Sherlock Singler" due to his track record of capturing criminals. Singler introduced fingerprinting to southern Oregon after learning the technique while in Sacramento extraditing a prisoner. Singler was the first law enforcement officer in southern Oregon to use bloodhounds to track criminals. In 1912, Singler was elected county sheriff. He took office on January 7, 1913, and moved his wife and eight children to Jacksonville. His wife worked cooking meals for the prisoners at the Jacksonville jail. Singler had only been on the job four months when he received word that Lester Jones had returned to Jacksonville. Jones was one of Jackson County's most wanted criminals. Armed with an arrest warrant and a gun, Singler approached the cabin where Jones was staying. Singler was immediately met with gunfire. Although two shots went into his lungs, he was able to return fire and killed Jones instantly. Sheriff Singler succumbed to his injuries the next day, leaving his wife and eight small children.

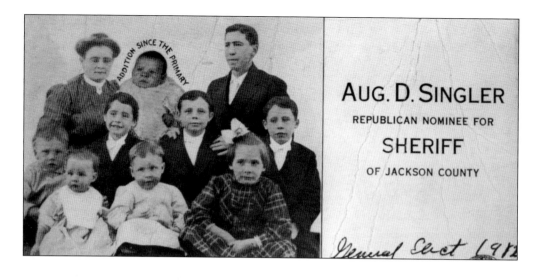

When August Singler decided to run for Jackson County sheriff in 1912, he wanted to make it clear to the voters that he was not affiliated with any political party. He had the photograph shown above taken with the caption that read, "The Party I Am Working For." The first campaign photograph showed him with his wife and seven children. Before the election, he updated the photograph with a new picture showing the addition of a baby to the family. The photograph shown below is of the funeral procession through Medford on its way to the Eastwood cemetery where Sheriff Singler was laid to rest.

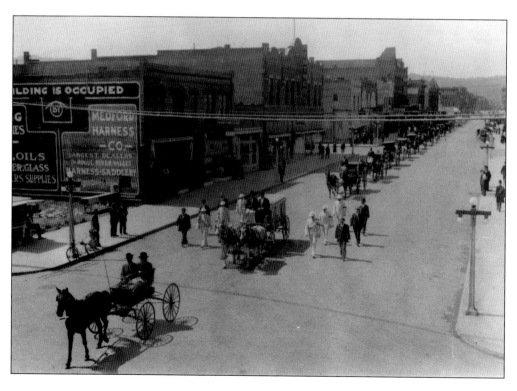

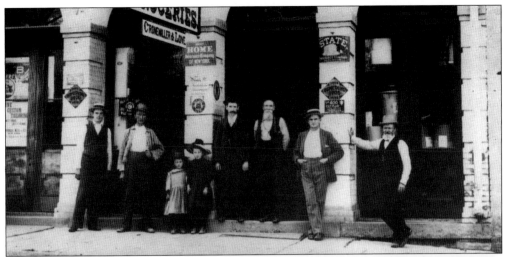

The men in these pictures seem to be enjoying a little free time in downtown Jacksonville. The dog and the children do not seem to be enjoying themselves quite as much.

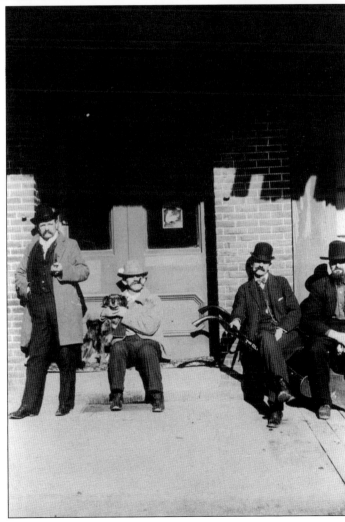

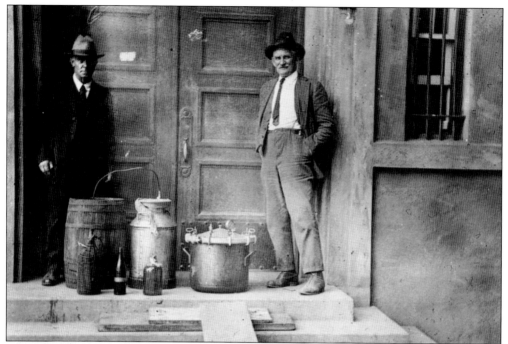

Prohibition hit many towns across America hard and Jacksonville was no exception. Pictured above are Sherriff Terrill (left) and L. D. Farncrooh with numerous confiscated stills.

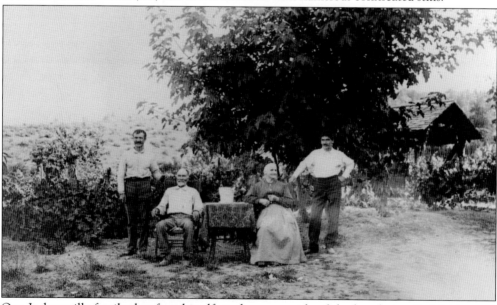

One Jacksonville family that found itself on the wrong side of the law during Prohibition was Auguste Petard, his wife Marie, and their two sons. They had immigrated from Italy and started a vineyard on the outskirts of Jacksonville. They were in shock when the Volstead Act was passed. Soon the sheriff showed up at their door and confiscated more than 600 gallons of wine. A court order was issued stating that the wine had to be destroyed. A few days later, the wine, with an estimated value of $4,000, was poured out near the Jacksonville School. Auguste was fined $75 and sentenced to 30 days in jail, which was suspended.

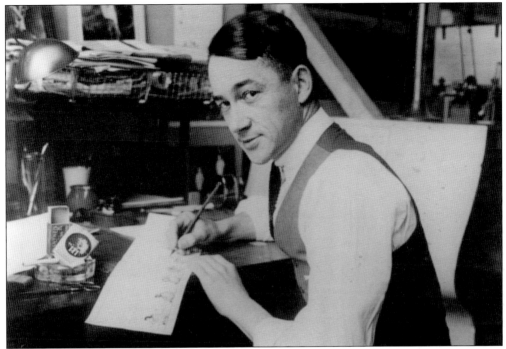

One of Jacksonville's most famous residents was Vance DeBar "Pinto" Colvig. Pinto grew up in Jacksonville, and made quite a name for himself in Hollywood. He got his start as a newspaper cartoonist and writer before joining the A. G. Barnes Circus and becoming a clown. In the 1920s, Pinto began working in Hollywood as a writer and comedian for silent comedies. From there, he went to work for Walt Disney, a career that made him famous. Pinto is credited with creating the Bozo the Clown character. He was also the voice of Goofy, Grumpy, Sleepy, Pluto, and one of the three pigs. Vance was one of Walt Disney's top artists. After that career, Pinto moved to Florida to lend his voice to such radio shows as *Amos and Andy*, *Maxwell the Cat*, and the *Jack Benny Show*.

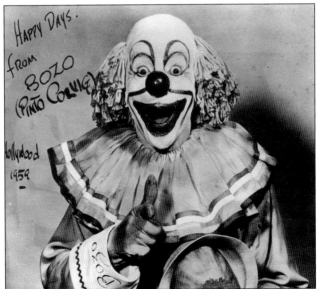

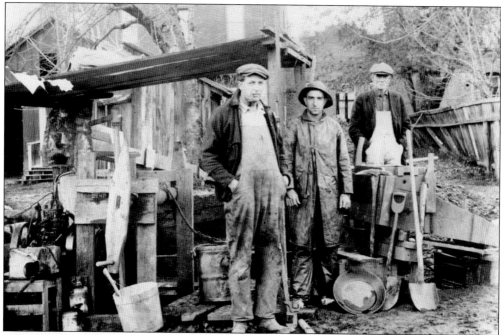

The Great Depression hit the small town of Jacksonville quite hard. There were so few businesses or employment opportunities in the town, that by then had all but been forgotten. Many of the residents of Jacksonville had grown up hearing of the gold strikes in the nearby creeks and surrounding hills. Faced with hunger and little opportunity, residents of the old gold mining town took to digging for gold right in their backyards. Others created more elaborate mining operations such as the setup pictured below. That particular operation is said to have brought in $40,000 worth of gold. All was fine for a while and people were enjoying their new found source of money, but then the streets began to cave in from all the digging and everyone was ordered to stop mining for gold.

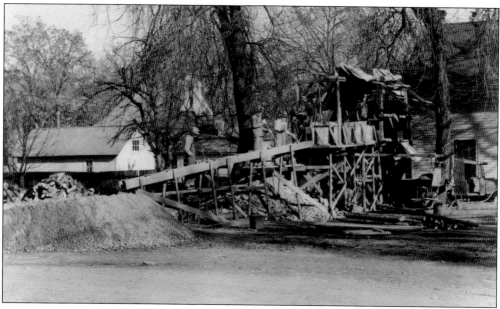

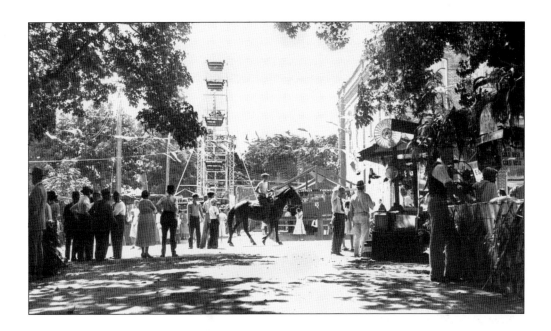

The Gold Rush Jubilee held in August 1933 brought the townsfolk together for the first celebration in quite a while. Times were difficult, and the townsfolk were in need of a reason to celebrate. A carnival was set up on Oregon and California Streets. The locals were asked to bring artifacts from the pioneer and/or Native American eras to display. People brought in items that had been passed down through the generations that had come overland. Other people brought in items from the Native Americans that had been found on their land such as mortar and pestles. The Gold Rush Jubilee proved to be a popular event and continued for many years. They were not held on a regular basis, but pictured below is a Gold Rush Jubilee from 1949.

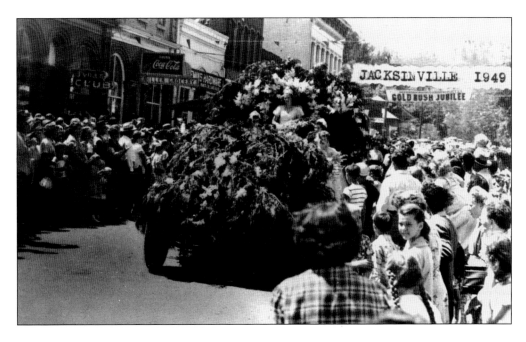

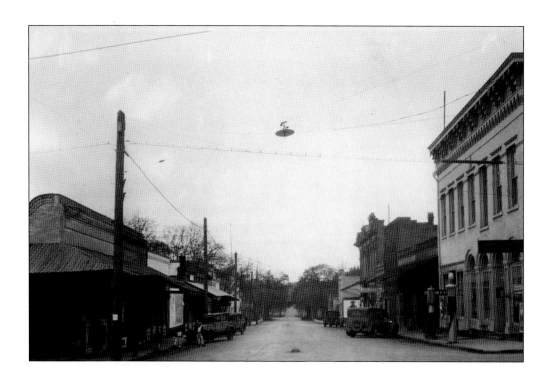

Even though there are a few cars pictured here, there does not seem to be much activity in the old town of Jacksonville. By the time these photos were taken, the county seat had moved to Medford and many businesses had closed. Jacksonville's population suffered as a result. It would be several decades before things would turn around for the old mining town.

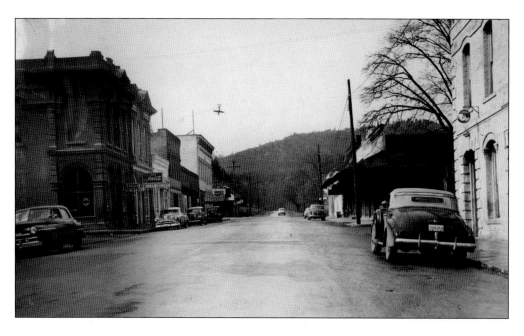

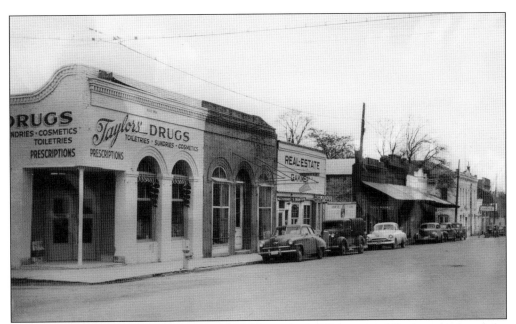

California Street has taken on an entirely different look. The automobiles have replaced the freight wagons, the mules, and the horse and buggies. An automobile mechanic has replaced the livery stable. There is a store that sells nothing but ice cream, something the pioneers could not have imagined. The items carried in the drugstore have changed and there is a real estate office, something else the pioneers could not have imagined.

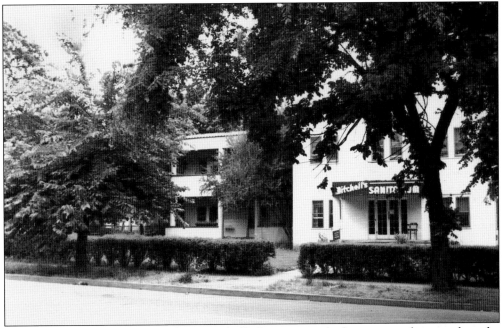

This photograph from the 1950s shows Mitchell's Sanitarium, which was across the street from the Jacksonville Museum. Beginning in the 1930s, Jackson County began placing the county's poor in buildings in Jacksonville. The value of property in Jacksonville was less than other locations, and there were plenty of workers.

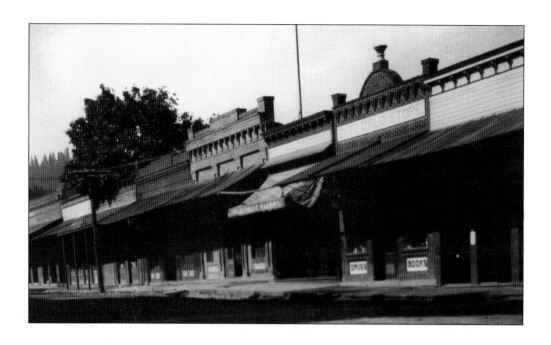

These photographs show a deserted town with several empty storefronts. Today those same buildings are bustling with activity.

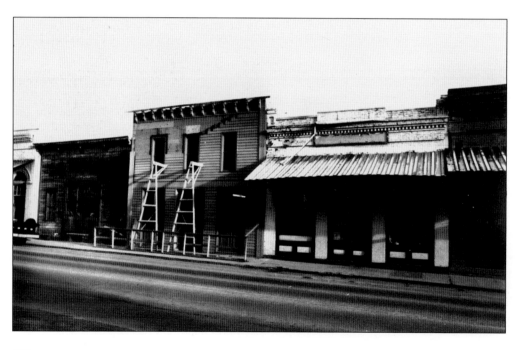

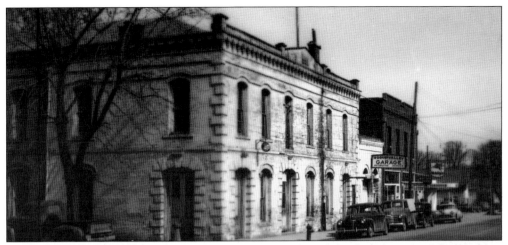

The U.S. Hotel building shown here is a far cry from its glory days when the townsfolk dressed in their finery and attended balls and parties that lasted until the early morning hours. In the 1940s, it housed a city museum. In 1967, the U.S. Hotel was the first building in town to be renovated.

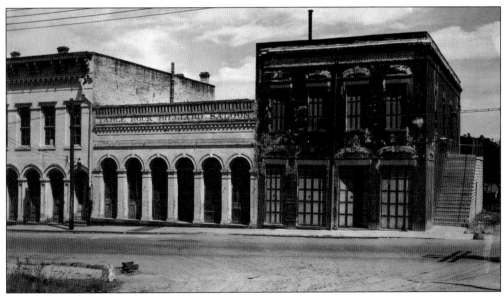

The Odd Fellows building, the Table Rock Saloon, and the Masonic building have fallen on hard times. Today all of these buildings have been restored and are an important part of Jacksonville.

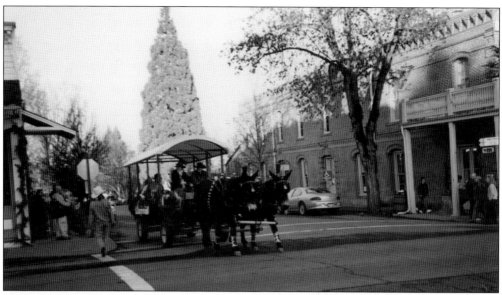

Today the town of Jacksonville is a thriving community where the locals walk to the local grocery store and the post office, stopping to greet one another along the way. Tourists and locals alike enjoy visiting downtown Jacksonville. There are no large box stores, no fast food chains, and the downtown looks much as it did 150 years ago.

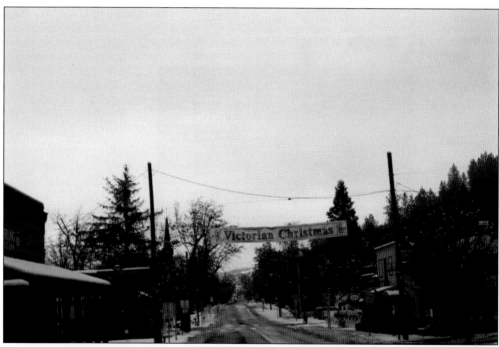

Every year, Jacksonville hosts a Victorian Christmas celebration. People come from near and far to visit with Father Christmas at the North Pole. They hear the latest news from the town crier while listening to the carolers in period costumes strolling the quaint streets of this very unique town.

About the Organization

All of the historic images in this book are part of the vast collection of the Southern Oregon Historical Society, one of the state's largest archives and repositories of late-19th century photographs of Pacific Northwest settlement. The Southern Oregon Historical Society was formed in 1946 in an effort to save the old Jacksonville Courthouse, built in Jacksonville in 1883. Twenty years had passed since the county seat moved to Medford and the building was in desperate need of repair. Windows were broken out, transients were sleeping in the building, and what was once known as the "Crowning Glory of Jacksonville" had become an abandoned relic of the past. The Southern Oregon Historical Society restored the Jacksonville Courthouse to its glory days and opened a museum in the building. Over the years, the collection grew and today the society is responsible for the preservation of over a quarter of a million artifacts and tens of thousands of documents and photographs. The Southern Oregon Historical Society is funded entirely by members and donors. To learn more or to become a member or make a donation, visit sohs.org or phone (541) 899-8123. You may also purchase copies of any of the historic photographs in this book by contacting the Southern Oregon Historical Society.

www.arcadiapublishing.com

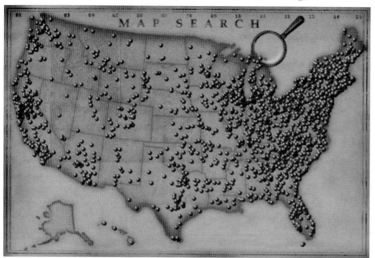

Discover books about the town where you grew up, the cities where your friends and families live, the town where your parents met, or even that retirement spot you've been dreaming about. Our Web site provides history lovers with exclusive deals, advanced notification about new titles, e-mail alerts of author events, and much more.

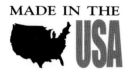

MADE IN THE USA

Arcadia Publishing, the leading local history publisher in the United States, is committed to making history accessible and meaningful through publishing books that celebrate and preserve the heritage of America's people and places. Consistent with our mission to preserve history on a local level, this book was printed in South Carolina on American-made paper and manufactured entirely in the United States.

This book carries the accredited Forest Stewardship Council (FSC) label and is printed on 100 percent FSC-certified paper. Products carrying the FSC label are independently certified to assure consumers that they come from forests that are managed to meet the social, economic, and ecological needs of present and future generations.

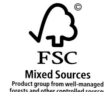

FSC
Mixed Sources
Product group from well-managed forests and other controlled sources

Cert no. SW-COC-001530
www.fsc.org
© 1996 Forest Stewardship Council

Find Your Place in History.